DEMONISED DOCTORING

DR. CHARL DU RANDT

IzakTheWriter

CONTENTS

Demonised Doctoring	v
The Satanic Plot	vii
About the Author	ix
-Foreword-	xi
Acknowledgments	xiii
Table Of Contents	1
Introduction	3
1. Defining the concepts	7
2. In the beginning	27
3. Rituals leading to hell	45
4. Engineering society for genocide	63
5. What is science?	81
6. Know the tree by it's fruit	105
7. Serial deception	153
8. Sinister Snippets	169
9. Control at all costs	199
10. Parting thoughts	225
11. Protecting Health	229
Glossary of terms and concepts	243
Index	247
Reference	257

DEMONISED DOCTORING

Exposing the occultic mission of the medical industry.

THE SATANIC PLOT

Also exposed is the satanic plot of the pharmaceutical/medical/industrial complex to foster control of humans, by robbing them of their health and free access to healing.

ABOUT THE AUTHOR

Dr. Charl du Randt

https://www.metabolewellness.com
support@metabolewellness.com

https://www.izak.blog
support@izak.blog

For more information visit Izak.Blog
https://www.metabolewellness.com
support@metabolewellness.com

- FOREWORD -

Having had the privilege of proof-reading this manuscript, I can assure the reader that he or she too is very privileged indeed to be availed of the opportunity to read this timeous book, aptly titled "Demonised Doctoring". Never has the time been more critical for an ailing humanity to be made more aware of the natural laws of health and healing, and to be warned of the hellish perils awaiting every unfortunate victim of the "medical system".

Contrary to the fraudulent media propaganda about miraculous surgical interventions, wonder drugs and high tech magic bullet diagnostic and treatment wizardry, the entire sector outside of casualty care is minimally a cutthroat business, accurately encapsulated by the term "medical industrial complex". To the rare few working with the Lord's divine guidance at the research interface between mirage and reality, as has my dear friend and colleague Dr. Charl du Randt, author of this book, an even more shocking picture is revealed.

As with any big business, the buck becomes the golden idol on which wholesome values are soon sacrificed for more money and power over both the consumer and the opposition. In the unique case of medicine, activities range from extremely rare philanthropy to very common mass poisoning; mechanical, radiation and chemical torture and mutilation, and eventually, usually murder, and all of this at a "bargain price in the service of humankind".

Medicine has a serious vested interest. It prospers at the perpetuation of human suffering. Bargains however become unaffordable virtually overnight when the patient's medical aid and other funds are exhausted, and they are abandoned to die from their medical wounds.

By no stretch of the imagination can the upper hierarchy steering the allopathic medical paradigm be deemed anything but evil, indeed the Devil itself is at the apex of its pyramid. Many exceedingly brave individuals have exposed aspects of this insidiously developing spectre over the past few decades. To mind comes Ivan Illich (Medical Nemesis), Eustace Mullins (Murder by Injection), Hans Ruesch (Naked Empress: The Great Medical Fraud), G Edward Griffin (World without Cancer), Lynne Mc Taggart (What Doctors Don't Tell You), Ralph Moss (The Cancer Industry) and James Carter (Racketeering in Medicine).

None of the above, nor their equally insightful, incensed and brave predecessors and contemporaries however, have so firmly taken the Beast by the horns as has our brother, Charl du Randt. Charl has stood by my side as a health freedom fighter and prayed for my protection as I challenged the shadow of the Beast by way of the South African Medicines Control Council as National Co-ordinator of PHARMAPACT, the Peoples Health Alliance Rejecting Medical Authoritarianism, Prejudice And Conspiratorial Tyranny, of which Charl is a regional representative.

ACKNOWLEDGMENTS

I now stand in awe as Charl du Randt launches this direct attack against the pulsating jugular vein of the Beast itself, the Medical Monolith, the Sword of the New World Order, preparatory to the Grim Reaper ushering in the apocalyptic end times. Charl du Randt is a modern day exorcist, holding the Light of Biblical Truth to the very face of Satan itself. This book deserves the widest possible distribution and we owe its author and his committed and supportive wife, a massive applause and our blessings for their dedication to this task.

Stuart Thomson,
Director,
The Gaia Research Institute,
Garden of Eden,
SOUTH AFRICA.

Many people normally contribute towards complex research projects, and this book enjoyed the sincere support and input of hundreds of patients, friends and scientists. Their role is acknowledged with gratitude and respect.

Critical to the initiation of the project however, were three parties in particular, without whose inspiration this book would never have even started. The first is my Lord Jesus Christ and His Spirit, whose amazing plan for my life has lead to joy, compassion and wisdom beyond my comprehension and most ambitious dreams. Secondly, my loving wife Malinda, whose understanding and caring wisdom inspired me to embark into the strange territory (for me) of book writing, and the dedication demanded of after-hours work. She had, on occasion, and thankfully so, resorted to severe cajoling tactics in order to keep me on track with this project. Thirdly, the dedicated support of the people at Metabole Clinic, under the astute leadership of Mrs. Ansie Cowley, made it possible for me to divide my attention between the running of a clinic and the part-time writing of a book.

Finally, Vic O'Kelly as publisher/printer and Dr. Leonie van Heerden as editor, have seen to the transition of the book from a manuscript to a polished product, fit for publication. Their teamwork, exceptional skills and professional wisdom have literally made the book available for all to see the truth.

Charl du Randt
   24 July 1999

TABLE OF CONTENTS

INTRODUCTION

CHAPTER 1: DEFINING THE CONCEPTS

CHAPTER 2: IN THE BEGINNING

CHAPTER 3: RITUALS LEADING TO HELL

CHAPTER 4: ENGINEERING SOCIETY FOR GENOCIDE

CHAPTER 5: WHAT IS SCIENCE?

CHAPTER 6: KNOW THE TREE BY ITS FRUIT

CHAPTER 7: SERIAL DECEPTION

CHAPTER 8: SINISTER SNIPPETS

CHAPTER 9: CONTROL AT ALL COSTS

CHAPTER 10: PARTING THOUGHTS

CHAPTER 11: PROTECTING HEALTH

GLOSSARY OF TERMS AND CONCEPTS

INDEX

ORDERING OF BOOKS

REFERENCE

COPYRIGHT

INTRODUCTION

"Be sober, be vigilant, because your adversary the devil, as a roaring lion, walketh about, seeking whom he may devour". (1 Peter 5:8) [1]

THIS BOOK IS WRITTEN in order to share information with fellow humans. Billions of people have been deceived, damaged, deprived of health, robbed of their possessions and murdered over the last 300 years, by means of so-called health care. The process is intensifying and is reaching a crescendo in the late nineties of this century. This brutal activity takes place under the guise of "health care" or medical treatment. The participants in this macabre scene consist of many stakeholders, including somewhat unwitting, normally willing, and innocent patients on the receiving end. Dispensing this mayhem is a multitude of professions, groups, academics, big business, government and the media. Once medical science is investigated in detail, one discovers that very little in the healing industry has evolved by chance, but that powerful influences have, and are, orchestrating the developments worldwide.

DISEASE AND ILLNESS have accompanied humans since the earliest history recorded in the Old Testament. In the first case of recorded healing, Abraham prayed to God for the healing of Abimelech, his wife and his maidservants, and they were healed. Health was, and still is also regarded as a blessing by believers and others. We know two factual characteristics of humans, namely that they are created as mortal, as well as self healing creatures – meaning that it is known from Scripture that humans are destined to die physically; it is also known from observation and experience that most injuries will heal spontaneously, without treatment intervention.

IN ORDER to fully understand the bigger picture of the medical puzzle, one requires a working knowledge of medicine, healing, disease, history, science, politics, economics, worldly traditions, and most of all, Scripture. The author has studied these subjects for more than 30 years. It was only in 1993 however, that he, by the grace of God, became saved as a born again Christian. Piece by piece the puzzle became clear to the author. Under the guidance of the Holy Spirit he devoted most of his free time to collating the necessary information for this book. The project has consumed 5 years of devoted work. Only a person, who has been a scholar of God's grand plan, as described in Scripture, can possibly comprehend the proper context of these worldly events. Having had personal experience of the Gestapo tactics practiced by the medical authorities, the author feels compelled to share his understanding and knowledge of the grave status quo, with fellow humans.

THE AUTHOR HAS DEVELOPED a burden of knowledge with respect to the "bigger picture" of disease manipulation in the world. Health manipulation cannot be understood in isolation from other global events, and is better understood once the global agenda of controlling forces is contemplated. This book is the author's way of sharing this knowledge with whomsoever can benefit from it. It is a gesture of love and compassion for fellow humans.

REVELATIONS by their very nature are controversial, and this book is expected to live up to the standard of an exposé. No offense is meant, although guilty parties may be offended by the truth.

THE MESSAGE of this book is loud and clear, since it has to compete for an audience with the sensational nature of modern media. The book is written for all to understand and does not intend to become an academic dust collector.

THE AUTHOR MANAGES his own health advisory clinic where information dispersal, networking with health professionals, provision of health products and apparatus, hosting of training workshops and provision of literature comprise the main activities. Over 15 000 people (as of 1998), have made use of the services provided by the clinic. Many of the clients have benefited to the extent that they have experienced inexpensive and safe solutions to their often-serious health problems. The experience gained from the vantage-point of having dealt with many disease conditions, has equipped the author with sufficient personal experience and knowledge to deal with the subject of health, as an authority.

MOST PEOPLE ARE SHOCKED when first confronted with the ghastly hidden picture of health control. Some of the best kept secrets of Satan are also shocking and can hardly be believed when one is first confronted with the diabolical nature of such events. Historical cases of massive genocide spring to mind as an analogy.

FOR THE COMFORT of the readers, the author deliberately uses language of a non-technical nature. Techno-buzz as well as the secret (occultic) language of the medical industry is purposefully avoided.

THE READER WILL BE ASTOUNDED and shocked as the full horror of the manipulative strategies employed by the pharmaceutical/medical/industrial complex are revealed.

BELIEVERS, as well as others employed in the medical industry, will find themselves regarding the dogma around them with a healthy "dosage" of discernment, after having read the evidence presented in this book.

After having read this book people who have been brainwashed by the propaganda machine of the pharmaceutical/medical/industrial complex will also better understand the allegations of occultism directed at the non-medical, holistic, or "alternative" camp of healing.

THE RUTHLESS DOMINATION of the precious health assets of humanity, by the pharmaceutical/ medical/industrial complex, will become clear to the reader.

THE TITLE of this book was deliberately chosen to indicate that the medical process of healing is demonised. It does not imply that all parties to the pharmaceutical/ medical/industrial complex are necessarily demonised. The author also distinguishes between demon possession, demon oppression and demonization.

FINALLY, the link between sinister plots of Satan and the pharmaceutical/medical/ industrial complex will become evident as the multitude of actors in this genocidal strategy are identified.

REFERENCES TO SCRIPTURE are taken from the Authorized King James Version of the Holy Bible, unless otherwise stated.

REFERENCES
   1 Genesis 21:17 (KJV).
   2 Hebrews 9:27 (KJV).

CHAPTER 1
DEFINING THE CONCEPTS

The medical industry is comfortable with the "absence of disease" as a concept of health. This means that in the absence of clinical evidence of disease, the patient is regarded as healthy. No matter how unwell, tired or ill the patient might feel, the doctor will pronounce that there is "nothing wrong" with the patient or that it is "all in the mind" of the patient. As long as there is no "clinical" evidence that there is some untoward statistical reading from the "pathological laboratory report", the results of the testing devices normally enjoy precedence over what the patient may feel. Patients are thus programmed to rely more on man made information devices than on the device God has provided them with, namely their God given senses. On the other hand the patient might feel well and hearty, but the technological pathology tests, may reveal that some readings are "dangerously" out of normal bounds and require "urgent" medical attention. This does not say that all information from a laboratory is false or inaccurate, merely that the reliance placed on man made information has taken on greater importance than those perfect and elegant warning signs designed by God, in the form of human senses. This principle states that one will know better than any device whether something in one's body is malfunctioning. The equipment and devices are sometimes useful as diagnostic tools used to determine the extent of malfunction, but technology cannot determine the difference between "health" or disease.

WHAT IS HEALTH?

Inquiring about the definition of health seems to elicit such a vast array of perceptions that one is tempted to think that "anything goes". At a recent seminar in Cape Town attended by 52 middle aged people, a survey was conducted by the author, asking only two questions namely

WHO THINKS THEY ARE HEALTHY?

WHO IS USING MEDICATION, prescription or otherwise?

ONLY ONE OF the 52 attendees thought she was not healthy. All 52 were using between 1 and 9 prescription medicines, plus some over the counter medicines as well! What a revelation. One wonders at what stage these people would regard themselves as unhealthy? Perhaps they perceive ill health only to occur once they are in a state of being bedridden, bleeding or in terrible pain. It is not uncommon to hear of people having a host of ailments such as arthritis, prostate problems and hormonal imbalances, complete with a history of two or more surgical experiences, and still regard themselves as being "healthy". These people are nothing less than "vertically ill", in other words, far from healthy but still alive. The origin of this strange perception of health does not exist in certain cultures, where any sign of malfunction or discomfort is regarded as ill health.

IT IS important to use an acceptable definition of health, since each reader perhaps has a personal definition, which may be in conflict with the theme of this book. The author has derived a general definition of health which reads as follows:

"**HEALTH IS a state of wellness which renders a person capable of performing all the physical, spiritual and mental, God given, functions intended for a particular person**".

THIS WOULD of course exclude those unholy or evil functions performed outside the will of God, and derived from the will of Satan and/or the will of humans. Other than bodily healing, a human or society may suffer from conditions which require, variously, the healing of: the soul, the land, backsliding, a broken heart, the water, hurt, empires and a nation. This indicates that any component of God's creation can deviate from standards created by God, and could then be corrected, or to use the Scriptural generic term, "healed".

FORTUNATELY, health is not a requirement for salvation. If it were, then the final stages of old age, which normally result in degenerative disease, would result in old sickly people losing their salvation! God is not subject to such silliness. Thus many believers may die due to disease, knowing that they are saved. However, wellbeing is an advantage when conducting the work of God, since sick people rarely have the zest and zeal demanded of God's workers. The proponents of the "signs and wonders" as well as the "name it and claim it" false doctrines have created much anguish in the hearts of their victims, by blaming the absence of healing on the victim! The rationale behind this false doctrine is that the "lack of faith" on the part of the sick person, is the obstacle in the way of healing.

THE MIRACULOUS MYSTERIES of the human body are beyond human grasp. One can only glorify God for the wonder of it all.

IN SUMMARY ONE can state that health is a spontaneous gift from God. Also that health can be lost due to many causes, and that it can be restored as easily as it has been lost, either by divine intervention or other means. If one is still alive, one can still be healed, since God's miracle of life abides in humans, and is active while there is life in one's body.

WHAT IS DISEASE?
    A definition of disease becomes as difficult or simple as one cares to make it. In terms of the previously stated definition -

"Health is a state of wellness which renders a person capable of performing all the physical, spiritual and mental, God given, functions intended for a particular person".

DISEASE WOULD THEN BE the loss of physical, spiritual or mental function as contemplated in the definition above.

FROM SCRIPTURE it is clear that, to quote F J Dakes:
"Sickness and disease were and still are special curses upon humans only when they will not obey or when they fail to understand God's provision along this line and do not appropriate it by faith".

THIS BOOK WILL UNFOLD the story and demonstrate how far humans, and in particular, the medical industry, have brought these special curses on humanity. Unfortunately, the holy servants of God suffer together with the unholy, because they are all subject to the same biochemical, mental and spiritual insults around them. To simplify the principle, one can use, as an example, the polluted air humans breathe in the cities. The city dwellers thus become "passive" victims of the air pollution, believers and unbelievers alike. Both groups suffer the same consequences because human bodies were designed by the same Creator, with similar physical characteristics. Humans are thus subject to the same physical vulnerability, believers and unbelievers alike. Humans have the promise from Christ that: "**The thief cometh not, but for to steal, and to kill, and to destroy: I am come that they might have life, and that they might have it more abundantly**". (John 10:10. (KJV)).

THE PROMISE STATES that Satan will steal from, kill and destroy humans unless they enjoy special protection.

ANOTHER WAY TO look at the issue of health is the phenomena that some of the healthiest groups of people or communities of people known today are not Christians, but, for instance, from other religions, such as the mainly Muslim living in the Hunza valley between Pakistan and China. The only disease reported from this community during the last 2300 years is childhood dysentery (severe diarrhea). Once past this hurdle they live easily into their 90's without any form of disease.[1] Could it be that their extraordinary health profile is due to their adherence to the laws of sanitation, hygiene, diet and the care of infectious diseases, as noted in the Old Testament of Scripture? The ninth healing covenant states it so clearly: "**And said, if thou wilt diligently hearken to the voice of the Lord thy God, and wilt do that which is right in his sight, and wilt give ear to his commandments, and keep all his statutes, I will put none of these diseases upon thee, which I have brought upon the Egyptians, for I am the Lord that healeth thee.**" (Exodus 15:26. (KJV)).

ALTHOUGH CHRIST DIED for the sins of all humans, the humans inhabit mortal bodies, subject to the biochemical laws of the Creator. Every moment billions of cells expire in a human body and are replaced with brand new ones. Inside the human bodies the death/new life process of cells is repeated billions of times per day. Even if one is saved by one's belief on Jesus Christ, and filled by the Holy Spirit, one's body can become just as sick as the body of an unbeliever, should one disregard the "maintenance" rules designed by God. Scripture not only directs one on matters of hygiene, marriage, children, society and food but also on the way to deal with animals, soil and the rest of the creation. Humans, as a society, have broken generally every health and other rule in Scripture, heavily directed by the medical-, food-, drug- and regulatory industries. Tragically, humans, as a group, are suffering the health consequences of not "hearkening", progressively and more severely, as time progresses.

A CERTAIN, often quoted, believer/medical doctor has highlighted the health hazards of not adhering to the rules stipulated in Scripture. He placed particular accent on the resultant effect of the spiritual/mental status of humans on their health. He enthused so much about these principles that his book is titled "None Of These Diseases"! With respect to his efforts of promoting Scripture, the medical brainwashing he has received from his profession is evident when the health hazards of medical treatment are clearly absent from the health advice contained in his book. Nutritional guidelines are also practically absent. He placed the accent mainly on the health hazards of breaking moral and spiritual laws of Scripture. One can only surmise that his intentions were honest but that the medical serpent had poisoned him to the extent that the book does not present a clear picture to other believers. One will certainly benefit by following the guidelines presented in his book, but the other major Scriptural health hazards have been understated, particularly the dietary laws recorded in Leviticus 11.

MECHANISMS OF HEALING

To understand the healing process it is useful to investigate the route by which healing takes place. Many classification systems exist and each modality will be driven by the framework or philosophy peculiar to that particular healing system. Underlying the healing process is of course the life giving dynamics as created by God.

UPON CONTEMPLATING the elegance and complexity of the human body, a famous British surgeon named Dr. Paul Brand, was moved to entitle his book on the human body :"Fearfully and Wonderfully Made", The book is based on Psalm 139:14. He was renowned for his charitable work and research amongst the leprosy sufferers in India. What it implies is that the working of the human body is barely understood by humans, and is of a complexity beyond human understanding.

LINUS PAULING, biochemist and two times Nobel prize winner, contended that each individual cell in the human body, of which there are billions, is more complex than a modern city.

HEALING PROCESSES CAN BE MYSTERIOUS, depending on the paradigm of the person who is contemplating the process. A small wound which is in the process of healing is a familiar phenomenon to all humans. By inquiring into the hundreds of healing modalities around the world (of which the author knows of more than 800) for each one's particular explanation of the healing phenomenon, the inquirer will be astounded by the vast number of different explanations. There is very little by way of agreement. The more "primitive" the adherent of a particular school of thought is, the more ethereal and spiritual the explanation will be. A native Indian may give credit to "good spirits" for the process. Modern scientist on the other hand, will credit "biochemistry" or one of many "rational", non-mysterious sounding theories.

SCIENTISTS TALK GLIBLY of living phenomena such as magnetism, enzymes, hormones, water and life as if these subjects are familiar to them. In the meantime, modern scientists don't even have the faintest idea how exactly these phenomena came about, or what exact roles they play, or how they function. At least the primitives admit that these mysterious phenomena are beyond human understanding and simply accept that supernatural issues are at stake. The modern scientist suffers under the illusion that these phenomena are understood, and so builds layer upon layer of explanation and rationalization on the false foundations of "science".

THE TRUTH IS that the only feasible explanation of life, and of healing as the restoration of life, is found in the mystical world of God and His Word. The best one can do is to "hearken" to the word of God, to observe the processes created by God with respect, and to promote matters the way God intended for them. Modern thinkers who have perceived the truth underlying some of these phenomena, have generally been ostracized and censored by the dogma ruling the establishment. This should come as no surprise to believers, since the Truth about God and salvation has been suppressed for as long as humans have existed. The concepts around "fundamental" and "absolute" have been stigmatized by the philosophy of the world, contradicting the very basis of God as having absolute and fundamental principles for humans in His Word.

SPONTANEOUS or automatic healing can take place only once the physical, social, mental, spiritual and ecological environments are in a status ordained by God. Human effort to promote or invoke healing will only work if these prescribed environments are respected and reinstated, whether for an individual, society or the whole earth. Any other way of healing is artificial (a copy or artifact), and will result in a worsening of conditions in the long term.

DIVINE HEALING (AS OPPOSED to spontaneous or automatic healing) is a recurring event in Scripture, and normally God does it with a purpose other than the healing itself. It serves as a special lesson or demonstration by God, in most cases, to believers and non-believers alike. As an example of divine healing, in Acts, chapter 9, Tabitha was raised from the dead, "and many believed in the Lord" as a result.

SATAN CAN ALSO EFFECT HEALING, with a purpose to deceive the victim. This principle is demonstrated in the following Scripture : 2 Thessalonians 2:9 ; Revelations 16:14 ; Matthew 24:24 ; Matthew 7:21-23. (KJV).

BELIEVERS WHO REQUEST HEALING from God may find that they are not immediately healed, but led to information which in turn leads to spontaneous or automatic healing. This action is of course still divine, since the information was granted in response to prayer, and may otherwise not have been available.

THERE IS ALSO a potential dilemma when believers pray for healing, of a disease which was caused by the transgression of the created biochemical laws of God. As an example the disease may have been caused by the long term use of a narcotic such as coffee. What is God to do? Heal on request? Heal as a demonstration? Reverse His own created biochemical laws to favor the sick person? Help the person to stop the caffeine addiction? Lead the patient to the source of information which will help identify the cause, so that the patient may become educated? The author would like to think that God would help the prayerful believer by making the cause of the problem, namely caffeine addiction and poisoning, known via one of many different options.

DISEASE of any category can also be caused by Satanic intervention, in other words not simply because the physical, emotional, social, mental and ecological environments are not in a status ordained by God. Many of these demonic causes are recognized by correct discernment, and can lead to simple restoration of health, but sadly the solutions have been kept out of the reach of most communities.

"......AND **healing all that were oppressed of the devil........**".
  (Acts 10:38. (KJV)).

IN THESE CASES one enters the realms of so-called spiritual warfare. The symptoms of devil oppression may manifest as any disease, such as fits (epilepsy) or asthma. How would one know whether one is dealing with a disease resulting from a physical cause or spiritual cause? If it is not an obvious cause, for example as in a case of malnutrition, which is overtly obvious, then one could suspect spiritual causes. A discerning of spirits is required in such cases. Fortunately one of the gifts of the Holy Spirit is "discerning of spirits", which would enable a person so endowed with the ability to diagnose the cause.

TO SUMMARIZE, one can expect to experience spontaneous healing as a blessing simply given to us by God as part of the creation. The healing ability may be lost due to disobedience, or by divine purpose, or by Satanic malice. The book of Job demonstrates how Job became very ill without being directly personally responsible for his disease.

ALL THE MECHANISMS of health and healing processes are beyond human understanding. At best, one can in identify which factor is interfering with the spontaneous healing process (by diagnoses or discerning). Once the interfering factor is removed or reduced, the spontaneous healing process can be restored.

WHAT IS MEDICINE?

About as many perceptions about the concept of medicine exist, as there are concepts of health. To most people in the western world it means a substance used or ingested, or a treatment applied, to reduce illness. To the doctor it means the profession which he practices, hence the word "medical". The medicine man of the primitives would consider spiritism, omens, substances and even celestial bodies to be part of his repertoire of diagnostic and healing tools.

THE WORD(S) medicine(s) is only mentioned four times in Scripture. Two of the instances mention medicine as something of inferiority, (Jeremiah), the third is a prophetic reference to the leaves of trees which were to be used as medicine in the new world, (Ezekiel), and the fourth mention has a vague positive connotation where the effects of a "merry heart" are equated with that of a medicine (Proverbs). Of note is that the role of medicine in Scripture is almost nonexistent. Surely, if medicines were important for health and healing, one would expect God to have given guidelines regarding medicines, as He did for all other important matters of human life.

ONE WONDERS how the pharmaceutical industry has become one of the biggest industries on earth, if God did not think it important for the wellbeing of humans? Could it be that such a monstrous industry is dependent on disease for it's own wellbeing? This book sets out to prove just that. Human suffering and disease are of such critical importance to the continued profits of the pharmaceutical industry that it is in the interest of the industry to promote disease!

TERMINOLOGY
There is much confusion about the types of medicines used today. What is a herb? What is a drug? How does one classify an injection? Is a personality altering drug a healing agent? Can substances which poison a patient, be called a healing substance?

WHAT IS IN A NAME?

Controversy and confusion about the names of medicines are raging. Legislators are uncertain and journalist's flounder when they want to classify or describe a like- minded group of healers. What do alternative, complementary, holistic, natural, traditional, energetic, allopathic, eastern, western and other collective nouns mean?

INDIVIDUAL MODALITIES (of which approximately 800 have been listed worldwide), have identified themselves by indicating various classifications such as:

CLASSIFICATIONS: EXAMPLES
    philosophy: Ayurveda
    methodology: Aromatherapy
    principle: Homeopathy
    origin: Chinese medicine
    originator: Rife resonance
    substance: Herbalism
    function: Nutrition Science

MOST OF THE above mentioned classifications overlap one another, but all of them share a common theme, namely that of intending therapeutic health goals. Most of the modalities are complexes of evidence, beliefs, theories, culture, fact and hypotheses. The word "alternative" is confusing since it suggests that there is a "regular" regime as opposed to an "irregular" one. For the proponent of one paradigm, all other paradigms become "alternative". Likewise the word "complementary" suggests that one modality is the "main" one and all others are "supporting" the main one. "Natural" is another misnomer, since not all things natural are necessarily at home in a human body, for example high dose herbs used in certain therapeutic applications.

ANOTHER POPULAR SUGGESTION WOULD BE "ORTHOMOLECULAR", meaning anything which is right for the body and which normally occurs in human bodies. It is an unfriendly sounding word and not quite appropriate since many "friendly" healing modalities do not involve "normal" substances e.g.

ozone therapy. "Allopathic" also presents a problem since it means non-homeopathic or anti-disease. "Orthodox" also fails since the paradigm of the reviewer will determine what will qualify as orthodox , thus the eye of the beholder becomes the criterion.

"Traditional" also fails since the users of a particular medicine will determine whether a medicine belongs to their tradition or not.

The error of classification arises when one modality e.g. medical science, develops an umbrella term for all other healing modalities. There is no term which will fit all. A solution would be to call these all simply "medicine" or "health treatment" proceeded by the name e.g. "Chinese". Even "western" does not work because not all modern medicine is from the west, nor is eastern medicine inferior to other medicines. Perhaps the term "dangerous" versus "safe" medicine is the real criterion for the patient and that all modalities should be classified as safe or dangerous.

"Integrative" medicine and "holistic" medicine are two more attempts to categorize medicine. Both names fail, because medicine which restores function is found across the whole spectrum of medicines in use today, and so the terms could be claimed by all and any modality.

It is the well reasoned opinion of the author that the only workable criteria for the assessment of medicine would be:
 (a) Safety to the patient,
 (b) efficacy in the maintenance and restoration of God ordained function and
 (c) honesty of information.

Technical reference works on toxicology and pharmacology would of course still be required for the purposes of classification, also known as the "pharmacopoeia" of each modality.

SAFETY MEANS that the end should justify the means. As an example, the amputation of a leg is an extremely crippling and permanent procedure. However, it may be required to save a patient's life. That would justify the amputation if there were no other way. Conversely, treating mild infections with prescription antibiotics is NOT safe, nor justified.

EFFICACY MEANS that it should promote the patient's own healing ability back to optimal, or as close thereto as possible. It also means PROMOTING matters the way God ordained, with minimal disruption of normal processes.

HONESTY MEANS the medicine does not harbor unknowns, both to the patient and the health professional. A person who is obviously dying, and recognizes it, would be defrauded by expensive procedures which do nothing to comfort the patient or has no chance of saving the person. Heart bypass surgery, costing a fortune, on old sickly people, must rate as one of the worst forms of medical robbery.

ANY HEALING MEDICINE, procedure, test, hospitalization, approach or philosophy can be assessed by using these three simple criteria, namely: safety, efficacy and honesty.

WHATEVER AVENUE IS USED in the healing process, one can use the above criteria to make decisions about using the respective healing process. The lack of safety, gross inefficacy and blatant dishonesty of the medical industry will become evident as this book unfolds.

DR. GROSSINGER HAS IDENTIFIED 6 broad categories of medicine worldwide. Quoted from his book they are:
    1.Simple mechanical, surgical, and herbal techniques that formed the basis of tribal ethnomedicine (cultural and traditional medicine) and led (notably in

the Middle East and Asia) to the technological medicines of Neolithic (modern) civilization;

2. Diverse branches of shamanism, embracing psychic healing, symbolic and ritual healing, visualization, divination, sympathetic magic, and primitive psychoanalysis;

3. MANIPULATION, originating in the folk traditions of physical adjustment and palpation and giving rise to the outlaw sciences of chiropractic and osteopathy;

4. ELEMENTAL MEDICINE, specifically the pre-atomic and componential cosmologies that incubated therapeutic pantheons in India, Tibet, and China (including Ayurvedic medicine, Ne-Gung, acupuncture, and related fields).

5. SYMBOLIC MEDICINE, flowering finally in the formal system of psychoanalysis propounded by Sigmund Freud and transformed by Carl Jung and Wilhelm Reich; and

6. REINCARNATIONAL MEDICINE, proposing a karmic basis for disease and practiced through heterogeneous systems tapping disembodied spirits and energies as curative agents.

DOES THAT SEEM CONFUSING? It doesn't have to be. Simply apply the test of safety, efficacy and honesty to any one of these. Armchair guesswork would be flippant. So, before making a decision, the subject under review has to be studied in depth. It is worth the trouble and time if it concerns one's health. As an example, one can select any one of the philosophies mentioned above.

USE "DIVINATION" from paragraph 2 above as an example. Is it safe? Maybe it is physically safe. But Scripture issues warnings about divination and regards divination, or the art of mystic insight or fortune-telling as a forbidden heathen practice . Dakes indicates that divination attracts 16 negative statements in Scripture. One can clearly see that it is a spiritual risk, and therefore unsafe.

SECONDLY, what is the efficacy of divination? One can deduct from the long history of divination and the popularity of the practice, that it seems to work for some users.

THIRDLY, how honest is divination? The practitioners of divination generally state which method of divination they will use and the alleged benefits, by being candid about their trade. They also don't realize that they are dabbling in Scripturally forbidden practices. The practitioners seem honest, but the practice itself is not honest according to Scripture.

AFTER SUCH AN ASSESSMENT, the informed believer would be loathe to make use of divination. The unbeliever would not realize that it is dangerous territory and would unwittingly be spiritually endangered. The practice itself is dishonest since it is a spiritually deceptive and treacherous endeavor, created by Satan.

ONE CAN THUS ASSESS any modality simply with some research, and by application of those three simple questions or criteria.

WHAT IS OCCULTIC?

The favorite allegation directed at non-medical or "alternative" medicine, is that it is occultic. The source of these, sometimes false, allegations is investigated in chapter 7. In the Christian media, the enthusiastic exposure of the New Age movement has placed strong emphasis on the hidden dangers of so-called "new age medicine".

THE DICTIONARY MEANING of occult is "secret, mysterious, supernatural, esoteric knowledge, hidden from view".

The Scriptural connotations take a more narrow view of the occult and generally mean those heathen practices forbidden by Scripture. The practices identified in Scripture are enchantments (magic arts), witchcraft (dealing with spirits), sorcery (spirits and potions, from the Greek pharmakos), soothsaying (as in predicting), divination (mystical insight or fortune telling), wizardry (expert magician), necromancy (consulting the dead), magic (supernatural intervention), charm (casting spells), prognostication (foretelling by indications), observing times (keep magic timetable), astrology and stargazing (predicting and being guided by these signs). These practices are effective but require the intervention of demons called "familiar spirits", according to Scripture.

THESE SCRIPTURAL CRITERIA for the identification of occultic practices will be applied to the medical industry later in the book.

THE GENERAL PUBLIC (secular or worldly) perception is that a practice which is regarded as occultic is "evil".

BEFORE THE ADVENT of the microscope, people had already noticed the fact that diseases could be transmitted. Not knowing what caused the sickness, they invented their own rationale for the phenomenon and many blamed the transmission on "evil spirits". For them it was occult, or the unknown, which landed these illnesses on them. Today it is known that germs act as agents of some diseases, and one can ask a pathologist for the identity of the germ. One of the first medical doctors to correctly identify the phenomenon that germs were a factor in disease, was a nineteenth century specialist from Vienna by the name of Dr. Semmelweis. He insisted that the Biblical practice of washing hands be observed in his hospital wards. He was fired from his job as professor and discredited by his bosses, for his heresy, and committed suicide once his livelihood was gone. The story of Semmelweis proves that the intolerance of medical dogma is not new. (for purposes of clarity the author uses the word "dogma" to indicate powerfully protected opinions which lack proof).

WHAT IS NATURAL?

The concept of "natural" is probably more confusing than any other concept in healing. Should a hormone which is identical to a particular human hormone be regarded as natural if it is made in a hormone factory? What then if it is extracted from another human and then administered, and not made in a factory? Is it natural to place substances from one human into the body of another human? Are blood transfusions natural?

Is a banana natural if it has been genetically engineered, artificially fertilized, treated with pesticides, picked green, cold storaged for months, artificially ripened with gas and irradiated with radioactivity? That is the normal fare for a banana in the industrialized world.

As far as Scripture goes, the only natural practices are those ordained by God, as well as anything which is not in conflict with God's plans. How would one know what these plans and intentions are? From Scripture of course! A personal relationship with God will prevent one from being destroyed: "**My people are destroyed for lack of knowledge: because thou hast rejected knowledge, I will also reject thee, that thou shalt be no priest to me: seeing thou hast forgotten the law of thy God, I will also forget thy children**". (Hosea 4:6 (KJV)).

Technology is easily confused with the concept of natural/unnatural. Humans manufacture musical instruments which do not just "happen" in nature and cannot therefore be regarded as "natural" since it is a human technological innovation. Animals also build nests and beavers build dams, but they build these structures because God created them to do it that way. Also, each species builds only it's own requirements and no more; ants won't build birds nests for instance.

By using this Godly model, it now becomes easy to assess whether something is "natural" or not. Simply ask whether it is in conflict with God's ordinations!

Any subject under assessment for it's "natural" status may appear to be a complex subject, such as for instance the matter of water treatment by means of chlorine. Chlorine reduces germs (pathogens) in the water and may help reduce typhoid fever for instance, and the stated purpose of the scientists is to protect people from harm. At the same time the chlorine also poisons the people who drink the water. What now? The answer is that the safe ways of cleaning water and keeping it germ free, have been sidelined and suppressed by the pharmaceutical/medical/industrial complex. Victor Schauberger, the Austrian water specialist, already showed the world how water could be kept germ free, simply and almost cost free, as long ago as 1933. Ozone treatment is harmless and very cheap, but is hardly used other than in a few places in Europe.

So the question is simple and the answer is simple, namely that water and people are being poisoned with expensive chemicals because it was planned that way by the pharmaceutical/medical/industrial complex! Chlorinating is therefore not "natural" at all. To discover and understand this fact however, one has to lift several veils of spin control (indoctrination) which have been disseminated by the pharmaceutical/ medical/ industrial complex.

In summary, thorough investigation, contemplation, knowing Scripture, prayer and the guidance of the Holy Spirit, regarding any dubious matter, will reveal whether it is in conflict with God's plan, and thus "unnatural".

EVER HEARD OF ALLOPATHIC?
The terms allopathic, homeopathic, and naturopathic, are confusing to some people.

The word "–pathic" is derived from the Greek "pathos" meaning disease. The prefix "allo" means "opposite". Therefore an allopathic treatment would go against the disease, for example in an anti-cancer or anti-inflammatory medication. Most medical treatments are of the "allo" type where "war" is waged against disease.

"Homeo" means "the same", and is found mainly in the homeopathic school of thought. Homeopathy often treats disease with a remedy which can invoke the "same" symptoms that the patient is suffering from.

"Naturo" means "natural", and these medicines aim to use natural substances and methods, to promote health.

WHAT IS OPTIMAL?

Optimal health refers to a state where the health of a person is as "good as possible" or more "abundant" than they could imagine.

The definition of "as good as possible" varies from culture to culture. The medical industry have well defined (very early) ages at which one's health is supposed to go into decline. The expectation is thus created for a person to blame a host of illnesses on their "age" and the passage of time, never suspecting that there might be simple and cheap methods of reversing the illnesses. Other cultures, such as the Hunza, know that health is a free gift from God and that health need not be bought from the medical industry.

Treating the disease has become the norm, instead of health being treated. In the next chapter the reader will be informed of how the medical industry has it's beady eye fixed only on disease, and not on health!

References

1: Hoffman, Dr. Jay M. *Hunza, 15 Secrets of the world's healthiest and oldest living people.* (1979)

2: Dakes Annotated Reference Bible (KJV). *Page 566 column 4 note g. (1993).*

3: Dakes Annotated Reference Bible (KJV). *Page 80 column 4 note f. (1993).*

4: Exodus 15:26. (KJV).

5: McMillen Dr. S. I. *None of theses diseases. 1994.*
6: John 10:10. (KJV).
7: Pauling, Linus. *How to live longer and feel better. 1987.*
8: Acts 10:38. (KJV)
9: 1 Corinthians 12:10. (KJV).
10: Strong, Dr. James. *Exhaustive concordance of the Bible. p 943. (1995)*
Proverbs 17:22; Ezekiel 47:12; Jeremiah 30:13 & 46:11. (KJV).
11: Grossinger, Dr. Richard. *Planet medicine modalities. p4-5. (1995).*
12: Dakes Annotated Reference Bible (KJV). *Page 75 column 1 note b. (1993).*
13: Becker, Dr. Robert O. *The body electric. Page 331. (1985)*
14: Romans 1:26. (KJV).
15: Hosea 4:6 (KJV).
16: Schauberger, Victor. Tranlated by Callum Coates. *The Water Wizard. p 46-52. (1998)*
17: Altman, Nathanial. *Oxygen healing therapies. p28-30. (1995).*
18: Viebahn, Dr. Renate. *The use of Ozone in medicine. P 16-17. (1994).*
19: Brand, Dr. Paul and Philip Yancey. *Fearfully and Wonderfully Made. (1987)*

CHAPTER 2
IN THE BEGINNING

"Professing themselves to be wise, they became fools...."(Romans 1:22.)

"WHO CHANGED the truth of God into a lie, and worshipped and served the creature more than the Creator..."
(Romans 1:25.)

"AND EVEN AS they did not like to retain God in their knowledge, <u>God gave them over</u> to a <u>reprobate</u> mind, to do those things which are not convenient; Being filled with all unrighteousness, fornication, wickedness, covetousness, malicious-ness; full of envy, murder, debate, <u>deceit</u>, malignity; whisperers, Backbiters, haters of God, despiteful, proud, boasters, <u>inventors of evil things</u>, disobedient to parents, <u>Without understanding</u>, covenant breakers, without natural affection, implacable, unmerciful: ...."(Romans 1:28-31.)

THE PUZZLE of the pharm-med-ind complex becomes much clearer once the historical developments are known. In the quotations mentioned above, the apostle Paul makes some general comments about the nature of humans.

Firstly, he points out that they think they are "wise" but instead they are fools. Secondly, he states that the error they make is worshipping nature (the creation), instead of the Creator.

THIRDLY, he gives an indication of what God does to humans if they elect to leave Him out of their equations. God, and not Satan, will see to it that they are given over to a "reprobate mind".

BY TRACING the history of the pharmaceutical/medical/industrial complex, it will become clear how God has been omitted from the industry by design. In chapter 6 the results of being given over to "reprobate" minds will be seen.

THE HISTORY of western medicine which follows, starting from the ancient Greeks to modern medicine, may not interest all readers. For ease of reference, a summary of conclusions is presented at the end of the chapter.

NATURAL MEDICINE IS OFTEN CRITICIZED for it's country of origin or the philosophies of it's originator. Similarly, it is only fair to trace the originators of western medicine.

DR. ROBERT O BECKER has performed such an accurate summary of the history of western medicine, that the author summarizes it here, as a paraphrased rendition of Dr. Becker's account.

THE BEGINNINGS OF WESTERN MEDICINE: GREECE
(Emphasis and bracketed comments by author)

WESTERN MEDICINE BEGAN around 500 B.C. in ancient Greece, with the writings of Hippocrates. Even in those days "technology transfer" occurred, and the medical concepts of Chinese, Indo-Tibetan, and Mediterranean peoples had already found their way into Greek culture. Some 150 years before Hippocrates, Thales of Miletus, often considered the father of the groundwork for modern physics, "discovered" the lodestone and static electricity (from amber, called in Greek elektron). He proposed that living things were animated by a vital spirit and that this spirit was shared by the lodestone and by amber. Thales said, "The magnet has soul because it attracts iron," and "All things are full of gods".

THESE CONCEPTS WERE common to the ancient world and were probably learned by Thales during his studies in Egypt. However, his most important contribution was the philosophical idea that there were actual causes for all things, and that humans could discover these causes through the application of reason, logic and observation. This important concept can be the difference between the necromancer's dissection of an animal to determine the intention of the gods, and the philosopher's dissection of an animal to discover its anatomy and to learn how it worked. Thales of Miletus made the first step away from mythology toward the feeble beginnings of science.

HIPPOCRATES INCORPORATED many of Thales ideas into his philosophy of medicine. Hippocrates left an indelible stamp upon all further development of medicine with his prolific writings.

THE HIPPOCRATIC OATH was still in vogue until recently and is now being replaced by something less "archaic" (the same oath but a laundered version). Doctors were proud to take it when they graduated from medical schools.

IN MANY WAYS, Hippocrates can be considered to have been the "ideal" physician. . He was not arrogant or certain in his beliefs. One of the quotations attributed to him is: "Life is short and the Art long, the occasion fleeting, experience fallacious and difficult." Art in this quotation, refers to medicine. Hippocrates also realized that disease was not a single causal relationship between an external agent and a simple machine, but rather that each disease is the complex product of the agent and the body's reaction to it: "Disease is not an entity, but a fluctuating condition of the patient's body, a battle between the substance of the disease and the natural self-healing tendency of the body". These words of wisdom have been largely forgotten by modern medicine.

WHILE BELIEVING THAT A "VITAL SPIRIT" was responsible for "life" Hippocrates thought that it acted through four "humors", blood, phlegm, yellow bile, and black bile. Disease was thought to be produced by an imbalance among these humors, a concept very similar to the Chinese chi, or life force, which acts through the balance of yang and yin. His treatments for diseases included the use of many natural herbs whose properties were known through pre-existing medical knowledge.

HIPPOCRATES ADOPTED the ancient use of magnet therapy. In that event, "fire" is translated as the equally ancient art of moxibustion (a method whereby heat and/or suction is applied to acupuncture points on the body of the patient). Given this history, the old common thread of a vital spirit expressing itself through balanced energy flow and alterable by the application of natural forces becomes plainly evident in Hippocrates' writings. One of Hippocrates' achievements was the idea of the "medical school," wherein prospective physicians could learn their art and craft. He founded many such schools, or aesculapiae. throughout the Eastern Mediterranean.

TWO HUNDRED YEARS AFTER HIPPOCRATES' death, the aesculapea at Alexandria, Egypt, produced a remarkable physician and scientist, Erasistratus, who was probably the first man to scientifically dissect the human body. He discarded Hippocrates' theory of humors and linked disease with the abnormalities of internal organs he found by dissection. Erasistratus properly identified motor and sensory nerves and traced them to the brain, which he believed was the seat of the mind and soul (rather than the heart, as Hippocrates had proposed). He also described the function of the heart as a pump for the blood. While he described the "mechanics" of the body, he was a vitalist who believed that the life force was a subtle vapor he called pneuma. In many ways, Erasistratus was far ahead of his time. Had his ideas, which were essentially correct, gained acceptance, medical and biological knowledge would have progressed far more rapidly than it did. Unfortunately, his observations and ideas persisted for only a few hundred years, and were then totally swept away by a graduate from a medical school at Pergamon. That graduate's name, Galen, is well known even now.

GALEN WAS, in most respects, the antithesis of Hippocrates. He was absolutely sure of himself and his beliefs, arrogant, self-serving, and prone to falsehood if it served his purposes. (The reader will note the the similarity to what exists today).Wise enough not to directly challenge the great Hippocrates, Galen endorsed the concept of the four "humors" but added much additional material derived from his own observations and experiments. Most importantly, he proposed the attractive idea that for every disease there was a single cause and a single cure, which was eagerly adopted by physicians who, then as now, sought authoritarian infallibility. Galen was a prolific writer, and during his life he published a complete system of medicine, addressing anatomy, physiology, and therapeutics. This became the standard text and ultimately the dogma that dominated medicine for the next 1500 years. Unfortunately, Galen was wrong. His ideas about anatomy were incorrect, and his teachings on physiology were based upon falsified experiments.(this falsification process has never stopped since then). In his day his concepts were challenged by those physicians who were followers of Erasistratus. Galen responded with what can only be called a deliberate campaign of falsehoods and vilification. He "repeated" the experiments of Erasistratus and found them to be "incorrect". (and then called them "unproven) Actually, the opposite was true; Erasistratus was a careful experimenter and observer. However, Galen's dubious scientific integrity was never called into account, and no one bothered to repeat his experiments. While practically all the writings of Erasistratus were destroyed, Galen's writings have been well preserved. Galen succeeded by providing a comprehensive system of medicine mixed with pseudoscience that provided definite answers for both diseases and treatments. Though largely wrong, it carried a stamp of authority and effectively put a stop to any valid experimentation or questioning for the next 1500 years. Early attempts at logical observation by Erasistratus and the humanism of Hippocrates' "art" were both submerged by the false dogma of Galen. The first wrong turn had been taken. Authority and dogma overruled research and facts. Western civilization entered what historians have (for good reason) called the Dark Ages, in which medicine and science were totally authoritarian and included erroneous concepts of how the body worked. (Matters which have not improved much).

THE BEGINNINGS OF "SCIENTIFIC" MEDICINE

The emergence of Western civilization from the Dark Ages was primarily the result of one factor, the challenge to authority. In medicine and science, the first challenger was a man who was a strange mix of humanism, mysticism, early scientific logic, and a most abrasive personality. Paracelsus was the source of the legend of Dr. Faustus, who sold his soul to the devil in exchange for knowledge. Paracelsus had no respect for authority in any form. At the age of fourteen, he left home to wander across Europe and Asia, studying at many universities and, possibly, never graduating from any. His attitude toward organized learning is best illustrated by his statement that "the universities do not teach all things, so a doctor must seek out old wives, gypsies, sorcerers, wandering tribes, old robbers, and such outlaws and take lessons from them. Knowledge is experience."

PARACELSUS DETESTED Galen as an absolute fraud. He once burned Galen's books in front of the university before a "cheering throng of medical students." He stressed the fact that the body can heal itself, while the most that Galen's medicine could do was delay healing or produce disastrous complications. (it sounds familiar, doesn't it?) Paracelsus foreshadowed antibiotics by correctly showing that mercury could cure syphilis. He accurately described the cause of thyroid goiter and he provided the basis for homeopathy by claiming that diseases could be cured by minute doses of "similar" - chemicals that produced the same symptoms.

IN THE FIRST environmental medicine study, Paracelsus correctly ascribed silicosis (a type of lung disease) in miners to inhalation of materials from the mine, rather than to punishment by mountain spirits. His experiments with herbal remedies and alchemy set the stage for the future growth of chemistry. And he made extensive use of the lodestone in his treatments.

This remarkable man even brushed aside the attacks of organized medicine (which existed then already) and science. His fame was great and his lectures (to which all citizens were invited) were filled to overflowing. His writings were remarkably influential, particularly his major work, the *Great Surgery Book*. Yet, he remained practically penniless throughout his lifetime.

Many of Paracelsus' beliefs and ideas appear mystical and, to some present-day reviewers, downright crazy. One of his most startling statements was this:

"To think is to act on the plane of thought, and if the thought is intense enough, it may produce an effect on the physical plane. It is very fortunate that few persons possess the power to make it act on the physical plane because there are few persons who never have any evil thoughts".

Evidently, Paracelsus believed that thoughts had a physical reality and could, "if intense enough", produce an action "on the physical plane." These concepts obviously relate directly to the present-day ideas of extrasensory perception, psychokinesis, and parapsychology. While never explicitly stating so, this passage may also be interpreted to mean that Paracelsus recognized the power of thought or conviction to heal (also called the placebo effect). Paracelsus was a vitalist who believed intensely in a life force he termed archaeus, which could be influenced by the mysterious action of the magnet. He managed to combine this mysticism with a remarkable insight into future biological knowledge.

HE SAID:
"**The power to see does not come from the eye, the power to hear does not come from the ear, nor the power to feel from the nerves; but it is the**

spirit of man that sees through the eye, hears with the ear, and feels by means of the nerves. Wisdom and reason and thought are not contained in the brain, but belong to the invisible and universal spirit which feels through the heart and thinks by means of the brain."

SEVERAL CENTURIES before the rise of reductionism, (meaning the study of matter by investigating smaller and smaller sub-components of the matter, such as molecules, atoms and electrons etc.), Paracelsus saw the defect in reductionist philosophy and placed its future proponents among the "ignorant." Paracelsus built his system of medicine on the legacy of the life force, herbalism, and the therapeutic application of natural forces, which can be traced back through the Greeks to prehistoric man. Like Erasistratus, he trusted logical observation and experimentation; unlike Erasistratus, he succeeded in influencing the course of history. His legacy, derived from a visionary power, gave rise to all that we now call science.

IN A REMARKABLY PRESCIENT statement Paracelsus wrote that "the human body is vapor materialized by sunshine mixed with the life of the stars." Paracelsus died under mysterious circumstances at age forty eight, leaving his few possessions to the poor and his remaining manuscripts to a simple barber-surgeon.

THE SCIENTIFIC REVOLUTION GETS GOING

Two years after Paracelsus' death, Andreas Versalius, a military surgeon, published the first really accurate anatomical text, *De humani corporus fabrica* (The fabric of the human body). This work finally, and completely, dispelled the dogma of Galen's infallibility. The age of science and reason had begun. People began to learn about the science of living things (biology) and the science of non-living things (physics). The mysterious natural forces of electricity and magnetism gradually began to be understood. A few great scientists contributed the basic concepts and provided the foundation upon which the rest of science built its edifices. The first of these was William Gilbert, physician to Queen Elizabeth 1 and the first true scientist whose interest lay not only in medicine but also in the forces of electricity and magnetism. His publication in 1600 of *De magnete* (The magnet) clearly delineated electricity and magnetism as separate forces, established the rules of action for each force, and described the Earth as a large magnet. No longer was it believed that the compass needle points due north because of mysterious rays from the North Star! Gilbert's most important contribution was, in the tradition of Hippocrates, Erasistratus, and Paracelsus, a plea for "trustworthy experiments and demonstrated arguments" to replace "the probable guesses and opinions of the ordinary professors of philosophy." This plea was later expanded and codified by Francis Bacon in The Scientific Method.

DURING THE 1600'S, several means of storing electrical "fluid" were discovered, and better methods of generating static electricity were devised. However, knowledge of electricity was limited to static electricity - the same type as that is produced by rubbing amber with fur, or by walking across a rug. Knowledge of how living things actually worked also advanced at this time, particularly with the discovery that nerves transmit sensory information and cause muscle contraction. The brain became firmly identified as the seat of thinking and memory. With this knowledge came increasing controversy between the mechanists, who viewed living organisms as complex machines that are completely understandable by means of physical principles, and the vitalists, who believed in the mysterious, unknowable life force. (God). However, even among the mechanists there was apparent reluctance to completely exclude the mystery. René Descartes, the main proponent of the mechanistic model, still postulated a "soul" which he conveniently located in the pineal gland (a curious, pinecone-shaped structure located in the center of the head).

MESMER, UNDER THE INFLUENCE OF PARACELSUS' teachings, proposed that living things generated universal forces that they could transmit to others through "animal magnetism". He began treating a variety of ills using magnetic therapy. Because he was remarkably successful, he incurred the wrath of the medical establishment. (Things have not changed much since then). The orthodox physicians claimed that he was practicing magic, and in 1784 King Louis XVI was forced to appoint a commission to investigate him.

The commission's report was "unfavorable", ascribing Mesmer's successful results to simple suggestion. The only remaining legacy of his work is the term mesmerism, a synonym for hypnosis. Hahnemann, building on Paracelsus' "Law of Similars," constructed a complex system of medicine known as "Homeopathy". This system was based upon the administration of minute doses of the "essences" of substances that produced symptoms similar to those from which the patient was suffering. Hahnemann postulated that these essences reacted with the energetic vital spirit of the body in a manner similar to that of the lodestone, a treatment method he also advocated.

THROUGHOUT THIS PERIOD of scientific excitement, the argument between the mechanists and the vitalists heated up, with the vitalists eagerly embracing electricity as the scientific life force. In doing so, however, they were putting all their eggs in one basket, for if electricity were ever totally excluded from life processes, they would have lost the battle. In the late 1700's another remarkable physician, Luigi Galvani, stepped into this controversy. While he was a thorough humanistic physician in the Hippocratic tradition, Galvani was also caught up in the fervor of the scientific experimentation of the time. He established his own laboratory, complete with the latest instruments for generating sparks of static electricity by friction. He was searching for proof of the electrical nature of the life force, and he believed that he had found it when he observed muscles contracting when they were connected to the spinal cord with metallic wires. Galvani termed this " animal electricity," and he postulated that this electricity was produced by the living body itself. For some reason, he brushed aside the fact that this effect could be produced only when two wires composed of different metals were used. Allesandro Volta, a physicist and a colleague of Galvani's, at first supported Galvani's observations. However, he then discovered that the electricity was actually produced by the junction between the two dissimilar metals, and that it was quite different from the single spark of static electricity. What Galvani had actually found was direct current, or continuously flowing electricity, a discovery that has shaped the world ever since. Volta's "pile" of dissimilar metals was the beginning of the storage battery and the possibility of continuous generation of large amounts of electricity. Galvani never publicly responded to Volta's critique. This was unfortunate, because he actually had shown "animal electricity" flowing from injured tissue; muscle contraction could be caused without the use of wires, simply by bringing the muscle into contact with the cut end of the spinal cord itself. This later became known as the "current of injury", which is an electrical current found in any injured tissue. But by that time Galvani had been so discredited that the idea of the current of injury was relegated to the status of an unimportant curiosity. Galvani, like Paracelsus, was far ahead of his time. He observed and reported the transmission of electrical force across space, when a spark produced by his electrostatic machine caused the contraction of a muscle held with metallic forceps by an assistant across the room. This important principle remained "undiscovered" until Hertz's experiments 100 years later. Galvani even searched for variations in atmospheric electricity using antenna wires! Had he defended himself more vigorously against Volta's attacks and continued his observations, the path of science might have been very different. Fifty years after Galvani's experiments, Emil DuBois-Reymond discovered that the passage of the nerve impulse could be detected electrically. The vitalists celebrated the fact that electricity had again become the life force, acting through the brain and nerves. But this happy state did not last long. Within a year, Hermann von Helmholtz had electrically measured the speed of the nerve impulse and found it to be very much slower than that of electricity in a wire. He concluded that while the passage of the nerve impulse could be measured electrically, it was not actually the passage of a mass of electrical particles. In 1871, unhappy with this new status of electrical force, Julius Bernstein proposed an alternate chemical explanation for the nerve impulse. He believed that the ions (charged atoms of sodium, potassium, or chloride) inside the nerve cell differed from the outside tissue fluid, and that this difference resulted in the nerve-cell membrane's being electrically charged, or "polarized." In Bernstein's view, the nerve impulse was a breakdown in this polarization that traveled down the nerve fiber, accompanied by the movement of these ions across the membrane. This, he believed, was what DuBois-Reymond had measured. The "Bernstein hypothesis" was eagerly accepted and has since been shown to be essentially correct, not only for nerve cells but for all cells of the body.

THE SUCCESS of the Bernstein hypothesis resulted in the dogmatic view that this type of electrical activity is the only type permitted in the body. In this view, direct electrical currents cannot exist either within the cell or outside it, and externally generated electrical currents (provided these are below levels causing shock or heat) cannot have any biological effect. The vitalists, banking on the mysterious electrical force, appeared to have lost the battle. While there is now no doubt that Bernstein was correct and that membrane polarization is the basis for the conduction of the nerve impulse, it did not necessarily follow that the nerve impulse is the only method of data transmission in the nerve, or that such membrane polarization is the only way that electricity can work in the body. Orthodox science, however, discarded such ideas as vitalism. (another major error)

By this time, the anatomists with their microscopes had found that the nerve did not actually contact the muscle, and that a space existed between it and the muscle, which came to be called the "synaptic gap." The vitalists were pushed into this small space and forced to postulate that the passage of the nerve impulse across the synaptic gap was electrical.

The argument remained unsettled until 1921, when physiologist Otto Lowei proved by experiment that transmission of the nerve impulse across the synaptic gap is also chemical. As a result of Lowei's experiment, all traces of electricity and magnetism were firmly excluded from any functional relationship with living things. Vitalism was finally dead. (Satan won that round, since the creation of God centers around vitalism)!

However, this triumph of science was still surrounded by a mystery. Lowei was still considered a professor at the university even though he was elderly and retired, and he often visited the physiology laboratory, telling the students about the strange events that had surrounded his successful experiment. He had, he said, been wrestling for some time with the problem of how to do the experiment. One night, he had a dream in which the exact way to do the experiment was revealed to him. Unfortunately, when he awoke he couldn't remember any details! The next night he had the same dream, but this time he remembered it all upon awakening. He immediately went to his lab, and in a few hours had successfully demonstrated the chemical nature of synaptic transmission. Lowei's dream ultimately led to his receiving the Nobel

Prize in 1936. In his visits to the physiology lab, he would caution the students that they did not know everything, that some mysteries still remained.

BY THE TURN of the century, the idea that medicine should be based totally on science had become popular. As a result, scientific medicine, based upon the chemical-mechanistic model was firmly established. Its conclusive proof of efficacy came in 1909, when Paul Ehrlich discovered that the cure for syphilis (venereal disease) lay in a specific arsenic compound. Erlich called this "magic bullet", a chemical specifically designed to seek out and destroy the bacterium that was its target. He further predicted that for the rest of the twentieth century, medicine would be characterized by the discovery of similar specific "magic bullets" for all diseases. As Ehrlich predicted, this concept has dominated modern medicine. The allure of the simplistic and infallible cure is as strong today as it was in Galen's time.

WHILE MEDICAL SCIENTISTS HAD "CONCLUSIVELY" shown that neither electricity nor magnetism played any role in living things, the physicists and engineers had not been idle. By the 1920's they believed they had learned all there was to learn about these two forces. People were already enjoying the luxury of electric lights, courtesy of Thomas Edison (and Nikola Tesla), and listening to the radio. They were able to generate, transmit, and use these forces, and understood their characteristics. A new world, based on science and technology, was dawning.

AT THAT TIME, it appeared to be firmly established that the only way an electrical current administered to the body could have any effect was if its strength were high enough to produce shock or burns. Electrical force below this level simply could not have any effect. Exposure to an electromagnetic field was even more biologically tenuous. The false reasoning went thus: If the field was steady-state (direct current, or unvarying with time), such as from a permanent magnet, it could exert a moving force only on structures or particles within the body that were themselves magnetic. Since no such magnetic material existed in the body, there could be no effect from DC magnetic fields. Furthermore, while time-varying (pulsing, or AC) magnetic fields could theoretically induce electrical currents within the conducting solutions of the body, these currents would be very much smaller than those required to produce shock or heat. So, again, there could be no effect. As for living organisms producing external magnetic fields, as Mesmer believed, the question was too ludicrous even to consider.

THE PHYSICISTS, biologists, and physicians were absolutely certain that the life force simply did not exist, and that all living things were simply chemical machines. They knew that life was simply the result of a chance, random event between chemicals, and that it would occur in a similar fashion wherever the circumstances were right. They knew that life was simply the result of a chance, random event between chemicals, and that it would occur in a similar fashion wherever the circumstances were right. They knew that for each disease there was a single cause and a single therapy, and that the only valid therapy was either surgical or chemical. Finally, they knew that the living organism was simply a collection of structures, which worked chemically and were integrated by means of the central nervous system, with no involvement of electricity or magnetism. Life had been reduced to chemical machinery.

THE SECOND WRONG turn had been taken. As will be seen, the new scientific revolution has shown that the whole of the body is more than the sum of its parts, that the ability of living things to heal themselves is far greater than the mechanists thought, and that electricity and magnetism are at the very basis of life.

THE TRIUMPH OF TECHNOLOGY

Ehrlich's belief that science would ultimately provide us with "magic bullets" that would cure each and every disease seemed to come true during and following the technological explosion of World War 2. The antibiotic, penicillin, revolutionized the practice of medicine and, more importantly, provided the hope that other chemical agents might be found that could selectively produce desired effects on cancer and other degenerative diseases. The discovery of DNA as the basis of heredity strengthened the Darwinian concept of random evolution, and it diminished the stature of human beings to that of simple machines controlled by the composition of their DNA base pairs. Advances in the understanding of the body's chemical processes and in surgical techniques, such as the use of artificial organs and living transplants, have nearly brought to fruition the dream of Dr. Frankenstein, the cobbling together of humans from separate parts. Science is now preparing to alter human genetic material to produce a "better" person. The idea that artificial organs are the same as, or even better than, those we were born with is common in the popular mind.

IN MANY WAYS, modern medicine has gone beyond scientific medicine to a new phase, that of technological medicine, based upon the applications of this technological revolution. At the same time, technology has become dominant in society and in our lives. Electromagnetism has become the "dynamo" of our civilization, and through its use for power and communications we have succeeded in changing our environment more radically than ever before. Since science had totally excluded electromagnetic forces from life, accepting the remarkable "advances" without even questioning their possible biological effects. The third wrong turn had been taken.

THIS TECHNOLOGICAL REVOLUTION, now forty years old, has begun to show its defects. The medicine it has produced is increasingly complex, expensive and inadequate. Magic bullets for anything, other than infectious diseases, have failed and science is facing a spectrum of new diseases against which technological medicine appears helpless. The mechanistic view of life has gradually been shown to be unable to provide satisfactory explanations for the basic functions of living things. Its proponents have confused the machinery of life with life itself, and in the process have managed to learn more and more about the machinery of life but less and less about life".

THE BIG PICTURE now reflected in the pharmaceutical/medical/industrial complex is one where only those things which measure up to the shallow understanding of mechanics and chemistry are accepted as real. The real basis of life has been carefully removed from the sciences. Satan has triumphed spectacularly in this area, by seducing scientists into relegating the unmeasurable to the realms of occultism. Like baying hounds, scientists and believers alike have been programmed to reduce that which does not measure up to the "scientific model" to the trash heap entitled "occult", "mystic", "psychic" or "new age". The fact that "occult", "mystic", "psychic" and "new age" deceptions DO exist and pose a real threat to humans, does not prevent these concepts from being used in deceptive arguments (as in Trojan horse strategies). By using the deceptive paradigm of "modern science" as a gold standard, any and all phenomena which fall outside it's shallow, man made boundaries, are banished to the surreal realms of the "unproven". The deceptive nature of science is described in another chapter.

THE HISTORY DEMONSTRATES how the complex scenario of today has developed over hundreds of years. Many role players have come and gone. Some were even on the right track, but they were overwhelmed by the majority who upheld the dogma. Everyone who wanted to uphold the fact that there was something other than evolution at work, was sidelined. Many "fools" (per Romans 1:22) had to steer the destiny of science, and many wrong turns had to be made, before medical science could become the horror show that it is today.

THROUGH THE PHILOSOPHIES of grand perception creators, and manipulative leaders such as Nicolas Copernicus, Francis Bacon and Johannes Kepler, it was ensured that <u>humans were robbed of the proud position as the central figure of God's creation</u>.[5] The long string of philosophers and scientists had seen to it that <u>"God was not retained in their knowledge"</u>.

IN SUMMARY, the 3 mysterious "wrong turns" mentioned above have served to lead medical science down the road of blinded deception in which it finds itself today.

FROM THE REST of this book it will become clear that human leaders are not the morons they sometimes appear to be, but that they enact a carefully orchestrated plan of Satan, as fully prophesied in God's word.

REFERENCES
1: Romans 1:22. (KJV).
2: Romans 1:25. (KJV).
3: Romans 1:28-31. (KJV).
4: Becker, Dr. Robert O. *Cross currents.* Page 13-26. (1990)
5: Capra, Dr. Fritjof. *The turning point. p28.* (1983).

CHAPTER 3
RITUALS LEADING TO HELL

"But I say unto you, Swear not at all; neither by heaven; for it is God's throne: Nor by the earth; for it is his footstool: neither by Jerusalem; for it is the city of the great King. Neither shalt thou swear by thy head, because thou canst not make one hair white or black. But let your communication be, Yea, yea; Nay, nay: for whatsoever is more than these cometh of evil." (Quoting Jesus Christ) (Matthew 5:34-37. (KJV)).

"Wherefore come out from among them, and be ye separate, saith the Lord, and touch not the unclean thing; and I will receive you." (2 Corinthians 6:17. (KJV)).

"And they shall teach my people the difference between the holy and profane, and cause them to discern between the unclean and the clean." (Ezekiel 44:23. (KJV)).

"And he spake unto the congregation, saying, Depart, I pray you, from the tents of these wicked men, and touch nothing of theirs, lest ye be consumed in all their sins." (Numbers 16:26 (KJV)).

"The <u>graven images</u> of their gods shall ye burn with fire: thou shalt not desire the silver or gold that is on them, nor take it unto thee, lest thou be snared therein: for it is an abomination to the LORD thy God. Neither shalt thou bring an <u>abomination</u> into thine house, lest thou be a <u>cursed</u> thing like it: but thou shalt utterly detest it, and thou shalt utterly abhor it; for it is a cursed thing." (Deuteronomy 7:25-26 (KJV)).

"Now the <u>serpent</u> was <u>more</u> subtle than any beast of the field which the LORD God had made." (Genesis 3:1 (KJV)).

"And when the <u>dragon</u> saw that he was cast unto the earth, he persecuted the woman which brought forth the man child. And to the woman were given two wings of a great eagle, that she might fly into the wilderness, into her place, where she is nourished for a time, and times, and half a time, from the face of the <u>serpent</u>." (Revelation 12:13-14 (KJV)).

The Scriptural information listed above has special bearing on the trap that medical people, and in particular, doctors have been seduced into. The tragedy is that the person so deceived is under a curse from God for committing the abomination. Not only that, but the offending person then becomes prone to the legal right of Satan to demonise that same offender.

And if a soul sin, and commit any of these things which are forbidden to be done by the commandments of the LORD; <u>though he wist it not</u>, yet is he guilty, and shall bear his iniquity. (Leviticus 5:17 (KJV)).

All doctors are compelled to take the Hippocratic oath, or a variation of it, before they become eligible to practice. Older doctors, in other words those who are now in controlling positions of the academic and administrative "control" bodies, all took the classical Hippocratic oath. For information, the following extracts from that oath are repeated here.

THE HIPPOCRATIC OATH

"I swear by Apollo Physician, by Asclepius, by Health, by Heal-all, and by the gods and goddesses, making them witnesses that I will carry out, according to my ability and judgement, this oath and this indenture: To regard my teacher (Satan according to the author) in this art as equal to my parents; to make him partner in my livelihood, and when he is in need of money to share mine with him; to consider his offspring equal to my brothers; to teach them this art, if they require to learn it, without fee or indenture; and to impart precept, oral instruction, and all the other learning. To my sons, to the sons of my teacher, and to pupils who have signed the indenture and sworn obedience to the physicians' Law, but to none other. (ie total rejection of God. author). I will use treatment to help the sick according to my ability and judgement, but I will never use it to injure or wrong them. I will not give poison to anyone though asked to do so, nor will I suggest such a plan. Similarly I will not give a pessary to a woman to cause abortion. But in purity and in holiness I will guard my life and my art. I will not use the knife either on sufferers from stone, but I will give place to such as are craftsmen therein. Into whatsoever houses I enter, I will do so to help the sick, keeping myself free from all international wrong doing and harm, especially from fornication with woman or man, bond or free. Whatsoever in the course of practice I see or hear (or even outside my practice in social intercourse) that ought never to be published abroad, I will not divulge, but consider such things to be holy secrets. Now if I keep this oath and break it not, may I enjoy honor, in my life and art, among all men for all time; but if I transgress and forswear myself, may the opposite befall me."

THIS OATH IS PROUDLY DISPLAYED in most consulting rooms. Why take an oath to gods? Do accountants and lawyers as a profession dedicate their families to a "teacher"? Does the reader see the plot? Every single doctor in western medicine has taken this oath, or something similar. Even the paramedics and peripheral services have to pay respects to the people who are bound under this oath! In chapter 6 the "fruit" of the curse will be illustrated. Only a Satanic ritual could be more blatant than this oath! Read the Hippocratic oath again and then read the Scripture verses quoted above.

THE LATEST VERSION of the oath, (simply the Hippocratic oath that has been "laundered") is taken by modern doctors, worldwide as follows:
(copies are freely available from medical schools and associations)

ADOPTED by the 2nd general Assembly of the World Medical Association, Geneva, Switzerland, September 1948; amended by the 22nd World Medical Assembly, Sydney, Australia, August 1968, and the 35th World Medical Assembly, Venice, Italy, October 1993.
(Emphasis and bracketed comments by author)

AT THE TIME of being admitted as a member of the medical profession: I solemnly pledge myself to consecrate my life to the service of humanity;

I will give to my teachers the respect and gratitude which is their due;

I will practice my profession with conscience and dignity; the health of my patient will be my first consideration;

I will respect the secrets which are confided in me, even after the patient has died;

I will maintain all the means in my power, the honor and noble traditions of the medical profession; my colleagues will be my brothers;

I will not permit considerations of religion, nationality, race, party politics or social standing to intervene between my duty and my patient;

I will maintain the utmost respect for human life, from its beginning, even under threat, and I will not use my medical knowledge contrary to the laws of humanity.

I make these promises solemnly, freely and upon my honor.

A SCRIPTURAL ANALYSIS of this oath reveals it to be a masterful recruitment, by Satanic forces, of fresh graduates, for the ranks of the damned. Normal professions like accountants need not take such vile oaths, since they simply render professional services, and do not have to perform blindly within a dogmatic medical religion, like doctors have to. Once a doctor, or any one else, turns from the Godly truth, then God turns their discernment into a delusion, so that they cannot see the truth:

"**AND FOR THIS cause God shall send them strong delusion, that they <u>should believe a lie</u>.**" (2 Thessalonians 2;11(KJV)).

AN ANALYSIS of the modern oath which is shown above, reveals the following facts about the dedication made by medics:

"solemnly pledge" means it is an oath.

"consecrate my life" means accepting another god.

"service of humanity" means secular humanism, the very basis of New Age religion.

"teachers" means the demonised tutors who took the same oath.

"respect the secrets" means non-transparency, a hallmark of the occult. (In "double-speak" it could be used as an excuse for protecting the privileged information of the patient).

"confided in me, after the patient has died" means don't witness against "brothers".

"noble traditions" means perpetuating the evil.

"will be my brothers" means an occultic blood bond.

"religion" means God's Word is unacceptable.

"laws of humanity" mean the laws of Satan.

"promises solemnly" means it is an oath.

"honor" means human honor, but not honor to God.

It is blatantly clear that the millions of medicals who have partaken of these two oaths have rejected God and His covenants. The implications will become clear as this chapter unfolds.

ONE OF THE most surprising aspects of demonisation is that people become blind to it, as if they are "not there". A blatant example is the serpent god logo, symbol of the pharmaceutical/medical/industrial complex, which is displayed with abandon and pride. This occultic, pagan edifice is advertised, carved, painted, woven, printed, imaged, displayed, promoted, in thousands of variations, and revered by the world at large. How blind can one be! It appears on ambulances, periodicals, hospitals, medical universities, stationery, bedding, curtains, uniforms, pens, gifts, medical instruments and anything that can be marked with a logo.

THE SERPENT, god logo, appears in many variations of the same theme.

THE FORMAL NAME given to this abomination is the "Cadeceus" or "Staff of Asclepius", the same god to whom the Hippocratic oath is made . Not happy with one serpent, some staffs have two serpents so as to keep the yin/yang fraternity happy. The two wings represent the wings of another god called Horus, and the staff represents the power over the Tree of Life, or in other words, power over the knowledge of good and evil!

THE INFANTILE MEDICAL apologies given for this blatant devil worship, is that it represents the brass snake as used for healing by Moses in Numbers 21:8-9. What nonsense! Even that brass snake of Moses was idolized by the Israelites at some stage, and the use of it was prohibited in Scripture:

"HE REMOVED THE HIGH PLACES, **and brake the images, and cut down the groves, and <u>brake in pieces</u> the <u>brasen serpent that Moses had made</u>: for unto those days the children of Israel did burn incense to it: and he called it Nehushtan.**"(2 Kings 18:4 (KJV)).

THE SAME SERPENT which is idolized by the western doctors is found in most of the occult world. Why? Because the serpent is the prime symbol of Satan! Christ is the universal lamb and Satan is the universal serpent in Scripture!

THE SYMBOL IS as old as humans. Any good reference book will divulge the occultic meanings and purpose of the cadeceus and the serpent or dragon. For instance: Kerykeion - The Roman caduceus. A herald's staff, originally a magic wand. Two SERPENTS are intertwined around its top, their heads facing one another. An attribute of Hermes (Mercury) in particular. Variously interpreted, sometimes as a Symbol of fertility, two serpents copulating over an erect phallus. Yet it must probably be, understood primarily as a symbol of balance. In alchemy, it is a symbol of the union of opposing forces.
(Emphasis and bracketed comments by author)

WHAT ABOUT SATAN AS A SERPENT?

Question: I think one of the great evidences against the authenticity of the Bible is its treatment of the serpent. In the Bible the serpent is the embodiment of evil whereas ancient myths and religions give exactly the opposite view. The Bible equates the serpent with the devil, but the most ancient religions, some of which are even practiced to the present time, almost universally identify the serpent as the Savior or at least as benevolent and to be worshiped. How can the Bible be true and at the same time be so much out of touch with what is clearly the common intuition of humanity?

RESPONSE: This is a fascinating subject, and its implications go beyond our ability to understand fully. There is no doubt that the Bible repeatedly identifies Satan both as the serpent and the dragon, not only in Genesis 3 but elsewhere. For example, " And the great dragon was cast out, that old serpent called the Devil and Satan, which deceiveth the whole world" (Revelation 12:9). In view of the usual human revulsion and fear of both dragons and serpents, one would think that Satan would do everything possible to deny such a connection, yet the opposite seems to be the case, for some strange reason. How intriguing it is that both are so closely associated with nearly all pagan religions! The dragon is found on thousands of temples throughout Asia, while the serpent permeates and even dominates the religions of India.

IN VIEW of the natural human revulsion for these creatures, this association could hardly be of human origin and would require another explanation. The biblical indication that Satan is the "god of this world" and thus the originator of all false religions would seem to offer that explanation. Furthermore, archaeologists and explorers continue to uncover ancient representations of a woman, a serpent, and a tree in close association, a connection which undoubtedly reflects the Genesis story of the temptation in the garden. Even today, one finds ancient Hindu temples deep in the jungles in northern India bearing centuries-old faded wall frescoes in which one can still make out the woman, serpent, and tree. When asked the meaning of these symbols, the villagers, who worship the serpent, explain that the serpent brought them salvation. (maybe this explains the affinity of the medical industry for using the red cross as a symbol, themselves being fake serpent saviors, they also want to replace the real cross with their version of the cross).

SERPENT WORSHIP EVERYWHERE

In the temples of ancient Egypt and Rome the body of the god Serapis was encircled by the coils of a great serpent. In Hinduism one of the three chief gods, Shiva, has serpents entwined in his hair. Yoga is symbolized as a raft made of cobras, and its goal is to awaken the kundalini power coiled at the base of the human spine in the form of a serpent. Numerous other examples could be given, from the plumed serpent Quetzalcoati, the Savior-god of the Mayas, to the annual snake dance of the Hopi Indians. One of the greatest authorities on the occult (himself a practitioner of occultism) has written:

SERPENT WORSHIP in some form permeated nearly all parts of the earth. The serpent mounds of the American Indian; the carved-stone snakes of Central and South America; the hooded cobras of India; Python, the great snake of the Greeks; the sacred serpents of the Druids; the Midgard snake of Scandinavia; the Nagas of Burma, Siam and Cambodia . . . the mystic serpent of Orpheus; the snakes at the oracle of Delphi . . . the sacred serpents preserved in the Egyptian temples; the Uraeus coiled upon the foreheads of the Pharaohs and priests - all these bear witness to the universal veneration in which the snake was held. . .

THE SERPENT IS........THE symbol and prototype of the Universal Savior, who redeems the world by giving creation the knowledge of itself. . . . It has long been viewed as the emblem of immortality . It is the symbol of reincarnation . . .

In Greek mythology a serpent was wrapped around the Orphic egg, the symbol of the cosmos. Likewise at Delphi, Greece (for centuries the location of the most sought-for and influential oracle of the ancient world, consulted by potentates from as far away as North Africa and Asia Minor), the three legs of the acular tripod in the inner shrine of the temple were intertwined with serpents. As one further example, consider the Greek and Roman god of medicine, Aesculapius, whose symbol was a serpent-entwined staff, from which the symbol of modern medicine, the caduceus, was derived. In the temples erected in his honor, Aesculapius was worshiped with snakes because of an ancient myth which said that he had received a healing herb at the mouth of a serpent. Here again we have the Genesis story perverted: The serpent is not the deceiver and destroyer but the Savior of mankind, replacing Jesus Christ. At graduation ceremonies of medical schools around the world, where prayers to the God of the Bible or to Jesus Christ would not be allowed, graduates, upon receiving their degree, repeat loudly in unison the Hippocratic oath. It begins, "I swear by Apollo, by Aesculapius, by Hygeia and Panacea, and by all the gods and goddesses."

(Emphasis and bracketed comments by author)

NOTICE how the Bible depiction of Satan as a serpent and dragon, the deceiver and destroyer of mankind, and then as the god of this world, who originates pagan religions, fits the model embraced by the medical industry.

NOT SATISFIED with having their own special brand of idolatry, the pharmaceutical/ medical/industrial complex then foists another abomination on the patient. That is the famous prescription sign, used worldwide and in multilingual format. The sign is the Rx.

THE SYMBOL IS USED for the instruction (prescription) of the doctor (priest/healer) to the sorcerer (pharmacist), to issue the patient with a magic healing potion.

FROM A MEDICAL INDUSTRY TEXTBOOK, this is how medical students are lulled into believing the lie by making the occult sound like a benign fairy tale:

(Emphasis and bracketed comments by author)

FROM THE MEDICINE man of ancient times to the medical man of today, the evolution presents a fascinating study. The line of advance is not always straight and obvious. Yet, no professional owes more to the long, ago past than does the doctor. To this day the mystic sign Rx adorns the top of his prescription. Its origin appears to go back some 5000 years and to be based on the legend of the Eye of Horus. The Egyptians used this magic eye as an amulet - to guard them against disease, suffering, and all manners of evil . . . Suffering had made Horus a healing god. As a child, he lost his vision after a vicious attack by Seth, demon of evil. The mother of Horus, Isis, hurriedly called Thoth, scribe and sage to the rescue. Thoth with his wisdom, promptly restored the eye and its powers. This led the Egyptians to revere the Eye of Horus as a symbol of godly protection and recovery.

DURING THE MIDDLE AGES, the Horus Eye reappeared in a new form resembling our numeral 4. Doctors and alchemists scribbled it on their prescriptions to invoke the benevolent assistance of Jupiter. Gradually, by slow transformation, the Jupiter sign changed to Rx . . . It is this late descendant of the Eye of Horus which serves to the present day as a link between ancient and modern medicine . . . a true symbol of the durability, strength and benevolence of the healing profession through the ages.

IF THIS IS NOT WITCHCRAFT, then what is! And parents think that their child is being taught "science" at medical school?

NOTICE that some more gods have entered the arena, namely Jupiter, Thoth and Isis.

FROM ANOTHER TEXTBOOK:
   Egyptian Medicine

WHEN THE NEW-FLEDGED DOCTOR, fresh from his course in twentieth century medical science, examines his first patient and writes his first prescription, he avows himself a neophyte of a pagan magical cult. He may not know it as he scribbles his instructions to dispense the latest antibiotic or the newest sulpha drug. But, at the top of his prescription, he writes Rx, just a Roman 'R' with a stroke through the foot - and in this act he invokes Horus, the bird-headed god of the Egyptians. It is modern science reinsuring itself!

OF COURSE, as a rational being, he will probably deny it. He will say that it is no more than the dog-latin of the medico – "R" for recipe, meaning "Take", just like the cook's 'recipe': Take four eggs. . . .' No, sir! As Sir William Osler pointed out, it is the 'Eye of Horus,' the Egyptian amulet dating back 5000 years.

(EMPHASIS AND BRACKETED comments by author)
In summary then, the doctor makes an oath to a god, invokes the spirit of Horus, instructs the sorcerer to prepare the medicines, and the patient gets healing! Science indeed?

THE ROLE of the pharmacist is critical because his function is to dispense the magic potions. The word pharmacy is derived from the Greek "pharmakos", meaning sorcerer. This function has been largely taken over by the pharmaceutical manufacturers, who pre-package the magic elixirs.

BY OBSERVING THE MODERN DOCTOR, one can detect the strong occultic flavor surfacing.

NOTE THE FOLLOWING practices when next fraternizing with doctors:
   1. Witchcraft (dealing with spirits),
   The reader has seen the Hippocratic oath and the serpent and the Rx. Does one need more evidence?
   2. Sorcery (spirits and potions, from the Greek pharmakos),
   Over 100 000 body altering chemical medicines exist. Most drugs also result in an altered state of consciousness.
   3. Soothsaying (as in predicting),
   "Oh, you will have to live with that condition".
   "There is nothing wrong with you, you'll be fine, it's all in your mind".

"Don't worry dear, we'll fix it with a minor surgery".
"We can cure cancer with modern medicine".
4. Divination (mystical insight or fortune telling),
"You have 3 weeks to live".
"Multiple sclerosis is incurable and progressive."
"Our tests prove positive"
"Your fetus test indicate Down's Syndrome, we suggest abortion".
5. Wizardry (expert magician),
"The specialist physician says your condition is genetic".
6. Necromancy (consulting the dead),
"The post mortem by the pathologist indicates a brain tumor".
7. Magic (supernatural intervention),
"We can avert a heart attack with this medication".
"Try this anti-depressant, it creates a feeling of well being".
8. Charm (casting spells),
"We'll give the patient a sugar pill for the placebo effect".
9. Prognostication (foretelling by indications),
"You need to take this blood pressure medication for as long as you live".
"Our prognosis for this cancer patient is poor".

THE IMPLICATIONS for the perpetrators of these abominable sins are grave indeed. It could cause them untold misery and lead fellow human beings to stray. The untold misery, vast deception, ruthless plundering, murderous practices and insatiable greed practiced by the pharmaceutical/medical/industrial complex is more understandable once one realizes that the whole industry is in the grip of Satan.

IF ONE CONFRONTS A DECEIVED, medically oriented person, such as a doctor, watch carefully how they manifest when confronted with the truth. The really saved person will reason with one. The deceived person will react with anger and arrogance, stating that the critic is "unscientific", "dangerous", "unproven", a "quack", "non-medical" or "not qualified" to speak on health, or some similar dismissive and derogatory attitude. If they react by manifesting in these terms, one may suspect that they are demonised. Satan (the lord of darkness) does not like being exposed or being challenged, and can manifest violently when confronted, similar to exorcism.

COUNTLESS CHRISTIAN AUTHORS have expressed the Scriptural understanding that by dabbling in Satan's ways humans are at risk of damnation and an eternity in hell.

BY DOWNPLAYING the role of the laws in Scripture, people are led to believe that hell is mystical or mythical.

BY IGNORING the word of God, people may attract curses upon themselves, their families and also future generations.

A CURSE, by dictionary definition, is:
  curse n: a prayer or invocation for harm or injury to come upon one; evil or misfortune that comes as if in response to imprecation or as retribution; a cause of great harm or misfortune.
  curse v: to use profanely insolent language against, blaspheme; to call upon divine or supernatural power to send injury upon; to execrate in fervent and often profane terms; to bring great evil upon, afflict.

(MERRIAM-WEBSTER'S COLLEGIATE DICTIONARY, Electronic Edition ~ 1994, 1995)

WHEN A CURSE IS PLACED on someone, the purpose is to cause injury or destruction, sometimes to the point of death.

WHY THEN ARE Christians still so defeated and afflicted by curses? The answer is ignorance. You can't fight a battle you don't see or know exists. You cannot defeat an enemy when you don't even know he is attacking you. God's Word says the following:

"My people are destroyed for lack of knowledge." (Hosea 4:6)

"Therefore my people have gone into captivity, because they have no knowledge; their honorable men are famished, and their multitude dried up with thirst. Therefore Sheol has enlarged itself and opened its mouth beyond measure." (Isaiah 5:13-14)

"For wisdom is a defense as money is a defense, But the excellence of knowledge is that wisdom gives life to those who have it." (Ecclesiastes 7-12)

"Lest Satan should take advantage of us; for we are not ignorant of his devices." (2 Corinthians 2:11)

"If a person sins, and commits any of these things which are forbidden to be done by the commandments of the LORD, though he does not know it, yet he is guilty and Shall bear his iniquities." (Leviticus 5-17)

"For it is a people of no understanding, therefore He who made them will not have mercy on them, and He who formed them will show them no favor." (Isaiah 27:11).

"Hear O earth! Behold, 1 will certainly bring calamity on this people; the fruit of their thoughts, because they have not heeded My words, nor My law, but rejected it." (Jeremiah 6:19)

"MY PEOPLE ARE DESTROYED for lack of knowledge. Because you have rejected knowledge, I also will reject you from being priest for Me; because you have forgotten the law of your God, I also will forget your children." (Hosea 4-6)

IF ONE DOES NOT READ, study and obey God's Word, then one is rejecting knowledge. The consequences of this sin are grave indeed. However, God is quick to forgive when one repents, and the Holy Spirit is there to help.

MILLIONS of faithful believers have become regular patrons and supporters of the medical industry. Some believers have been so deceived that they even rise to the defense of the medical industry, thereby joining forces with the devilish plot of the medical industry! Some believers have been so deceived by the grand lie, which states that only "scientific" medical modalities are acceptable, that they have become unwitting allies of Satan in the demonic strategy to eradicate real healing modalities from the earth. Of course not all of medical science is evil – only the evil component has been exposed in this book.

THIS BOOK DOES NOT SEEK to defend so-called "alternative" medicine, nor does it intend to promote "alternative" medicine. However, as later chapters will reveal, there is an abundance of safe, effective and non-occultic medicine and healing modalities available, outside the demonised realms of the pharmaceutical/ medical/industrial complex. These modalities have been systematically and ruthlessly suppressed, maligned and eradicated by the pharmaceutical/ medical/ industrial complex. The serpent has been busy seeing to it that the majority of people have been robbed of their freedom to choose God's way, including the freedom to choose the real God.

AS STATED in The Handbook for Spiritual Warfare "An unidentified cosmic being called the serpent introduces spiritual warfare into human experience".

READERS WISHING to make a study of the dangers of idolatry for the world at large, can read the classic "The Two Babylons". In his book, the horrible dangers of idolizing the serpent are spelled out in detail by Hislop.

"THOU SHALT not make unto thee any graven image, or any likeness *of any thing* that *is* in heaven above, or that *is* in the earth beneath, or that *is* in the water under the earth: Thou shalt not bow down thyself to them, nor serve them: for I the LORD thy God *am* a jealous God, visiting the iniquity of the fathers upon the children unto the third and fourth *generation* of them that hate me; And shewing mercy unto thousands of them that love me, and keep my commandments." (Exodus 20:4-6. (KJV)).

THE READER CAN SEE EXACTLY what the implications of the commandment above implies, namely that by idolizing images God may curse the future generations of the guilty party.

REFERENCES
   1. Matthew 5:34-37. (KJV).
   2. 2 Corinthians 6:17. (KJV).
   3. Ezekiel 44:23. (KJV).
   4. Numbers 16:26 (KJV).
   5. Genesis 3:1 (KJV).
   6. Revelation 12:13-14 (KJV).
   7. Leviticus 5:17 (KJV).
   8. 2 Thessalonians 2:11 (KJV).
   9. Udo Becker. *Encyclopedia of SYMBOLS. P 164. (1994).*
   10. Otto, Dr. L Bettman. *A pictorial history of medicine. P 91. (1956)*
   11. Calder, Ritchie. *Medicine and man. P 57. (1958)*
   12. Strong, Dr. James. *Exhaustive concordance of the Bible. p 95.(Greek) (1995)*
   13. Dakes Annotated Reference Bible (KJV). *Page 75 column 1 note b. (90+ on this subject). (1993.)*
   14. Randles, Pastor Bill. *Making war in the Heavenlies. Page 90-98. (1996)*
   15. Hunt, Dave. *In defense of faith. Pages 213-215. (1996)*
   16. Murphy, Dr. Ed. *The Handbook for Spiritual Warfare. Page 27. (1996)*
   17. Capra, Dr. Fritjof. *The turning point. p28 (1983).*

18. Leviticus 7:25-26 (KJV).
19. 2 Kings 18:4 (KJV).
20. Hislop, Rev. Alexander. *The Two Babylons. (1916).*
21. Exodus 20:4-6. (KJV).
22. Comfort, Ray. *Hell's best kept Secret. Page 19-26. (1989).*

CHAPTER 4
ENGINEERING SOCIETY FOR GENOCIDE

"For we wrestle not against flesh and blood, but against principalities, against powers, against the rulers of the darkness of this world, against spiritual wickedness in high *places.*"(Ephesians 6:11. (KJV)).

"THE DIFFERENCE between education and massacre, is that education is more thorough and takes longer."(quotation credited to Mark Twain)

"THE HEART IS deceitful above all *things*, and desperately wicked: who can know it? I the LORD search the heart, *I* try the reins, even to give every man according to his ways, *and* according to the fruit of his doings." (Jeremiah 17:9-10. (KJV)).

"AND FOR THIS cause God shall send them strong delusion, that they should believe a lie. That they all might be damned who believed not the truth, but had pleasure in unrighteousness." (2 Thessalonians 2:11-12. (KJV)).

IN THE PREVIOUS chapter it was demonstrated that the chief idol of the pharma-ceutical/medical/industrial complex is found in the serpent (Satan). It is of intriguing interest to study the manner in which the plan of the serpent has manifested in the physical world. The "man according to his ways, and according to the fruit of his doings" will be discussed in this chapter.

As a control group, it is useful throughout this book to uphold the accounting profession as a comparison or control group to the medical industry profession. Both professions have the following in common:

Worldwide services rendered
   Used by all large societies
   Globally agreed standards
   Used since the beginning of human history
   Links to Big Business
   Both are secular (worldly)
   Both depend on their clients for a livelihood.

Should one of them then display any extraordinary behavior, one can compare and ask why the other one has not done the same. Pilots for instance, could also serve as a control group of professionals, but they have not had centuries of time in which to organize themselves, aviation being a recent industry.

From the reasoning in the previous chapter it appears that accountants do not uphold a "belief system". They do not engage in occultic practices, or suppress opposition at all costs. They do adhere to a methodology which is called the "double entry" principle of keeping records. If outsiders can come up with something better, the accounting industry would welcome it. They accept criticism and are often charged in courts of law, in cases of contraventions. In other words they uphold a group of common interests, which although secular, have no special mission to serve the forces of darkness and evil. The same comparison could be made between Satanists and say, shipping agents – the Satanists have an evil mission whilst the shipping agents are simply "of this world".

THE FRONT LINE of the pharmaceutical/medical/industrial complex is the medical doctor in various guises. The professional doctor person may be occupied as a general practitioner, academic, politician, specialist, legislator, research scientist, media specialist, law enforcer, administrator, or involved in one of the many bodies such as associations, trusts, foundations, charities, or support organizations. Society is therefore permeated with the products of the medical industry dogma. In most countries it is impossible to place anything in the mainstream media, unless it supports the dogma. The reason being, that somewhere, in the media process, alarms sound if the dogma should be challenged. Society as a group is caught in a web of scientific censorship which can be as severe as political censorship in any politically oppressive country.

THE WAY in which this status was achieved, was done by means of a massive brainwashing campaign, second in intensity only to the efforts to promote the neo-evolution theory. In order to brainwash large groups of humans, a belief system has to be entrenched in their values. All religions are based on this methodology. Once the belief is established, it becomes "anathema" (banned by the church) to differ from it. Most eastern religions are quite enthusiastic to kill anyone who switches to "another" faith.

THE PHARMACEUTICAL/MEDICAL/INDUSTRIAL complex has organized it's dogma into a massive religion, by relentless media control and demonised possession of the medical universities and research centers.

DR. ROBERT S MENDELSOHN (MD), who has seen the light, has summarized the entrapment with great insight. He was at one time in the 70's :

ASSOCIATE PROFESSOR, Department of Preventive Medicine and Community

Health, Abraham Lincoln School of Medicine, University of Illinois; nationally syndicated columnist, 'The Peoples Doctor'. Medical Director, American International Hospital, Zion, Illinois; Formerly, National Director, Medical Consultation Service, Project Head Start; Formerly, Chairman, Medical Licensure Committee, State of Illinois.

IT IS clear that he had been through the medical mill, being a specialist gynecologist (doctor of female disease) as well as an obstetrician (doctor of the birth process).

HE WROTE a foreword in a book[3] which was published in 1978. Portions of his findings are repeated below:

AND THE GENERALIZATION is that the golden age of American medicine is over.

INDEED, the only way in which modern medicine can be understood is as **a religion** - the religion of a secular society that has **rejected its traditional value systems**. Modern medicine has at least ten of the essential components of a religion:
 1. **A belief system**, modern medical science, which can no more be validated than the proofs of other churches of the existence of God.
 2. A **priestly class**-the M.D.'s.
 3. **Temples**-the hospitals
 4. **Acolytes** and vestal maidens-nurses, social workers and para-professionals.
 5. Vestments reflecting **hierarchical status**-the color and length of M.D.s gowns signify their rank.
 6. A **rich princely class** supporting the church-drug companies, insurance companies and formula houses.
 7. A **confessional** - the history must be given truthfully to the physician.
 8. An **absolution** - the reassuring pat on the back – "you're fine, come back next year".

9. Selling **of indulgences** - the outrageous fees, likely to bring down this modern church just as it did the medieval church.

10. Similarity of language - I have confidence in my plumber ~ but "I have **faith** in my doctor". The doctor-patient relationship is "**sacred**".

ONCE MEDICINE IS REGARDED as no more than - and no less than a **religious system**, it can then be treated as such, and **compared with other religious healing systems**. Unfortunately, the religion of modern medicine proves to be worship of a god who fails to answer, who is powerless, and who, in fact, **deceives**. This of course, is the definition **of idolatry** and in the context of this all of modern medicine becomes understandable.

THE FALSE GOD of modern medicine even goes so far as to require, like his predecessor gods of heathen religions thousands of years ago, **child sacrifices**. The ancient **Moloch** of those idolatries demanded that parents, in order to insure successful crops, pass their children through physical fire. The modern Moloch similarly demands that parents pass chemical fire (heat-sterilized formula) through their children (and multiple vaccinations and antibiotics; author's comment). The purpose is similar - infant formula insures that mothers and fathers can both go to work to achieve sustenance and success. Scientific studies as well as historical evidence clearly prove the sacrifice of life and health resulting from infant formula compared to breast milk, and only the approval of the physician - priest enables mothers and fathers to equate cows' milk to human milk. Indeed were physicians to behave according to the standards of science and **honesty**, formula feeding a baby would doubtless be considered child abuse.

(Emphasis and bracketed comments by author)

ONE OF THE reasons for the poor acceptance of the western medical religion in the oriental countries was that the Orientals already had powerful religious belief systems. The western medical religion clashed with too many of their established beliefs, and to this day the western medical religion has a poor standing in, for instance, India and China.

Unlike in the orient, in the western world the pharmaceutical/medical/industrial complex had a powerful ally. Organized religion and big business have had a 2000 year long love affair in the western world. This horrendous relationship is well documented in a book called "A Woman Rides the Beast", by Dave Hunt. In this exposure of the global joint effort between governments (or their bosses, big business) and the church, to control the world, the diabolical recipe for global manipulation becomes clear.

THE WAY in which the perpetrators of the pharmaceutical/medical/industrial complex strategy went about their final stage of world dominion, was by coordinating it globally.

RESEARCHERS TEND to blame the Rockefeller cartels, and like minded interests, as the main driving force behind the plans of the pharmaceutical/medical/industrial complex.[5] Many more players are involved in this global criminal network, most of whom do not formulate strategy, but help as employees to translate the plans into action. Similarly, soldiers who take orders to perform the gassing of prisoners in a concentration camp, are "merely" taking orders from their superiors, failing which they will be punished. The architects or bosses of the grand strategies are driven by evil motives, being possessed of "wicked hearts".

SOME STUDIES OF THE "HARMONIZATION" process at universities have been conducted by various researchers over the last 50 years.

HERE IS ONE SUCH AN ACCOUNT:
   (Emphasis and bracketed comments by author)

THERE IS AN OLD SAYING: "He who pays the piper calls the tune". This is one of those eternal truths that exist - and always will exist - in business - in politics - and in education.

WE HAVE SEEN HOW. John D. Rockefeller captured the hearts of **Baptist ministers** with a mere $600,000 granted to Chicago University. What remains to be demonstrated is that he also captured control of the university. Within a year after the grant, Rockefeller's personal choice, Dr. William Rainey Harper was named president of the institution. And within two years, the **teaching staff had been successfully purged** of all anti-Rockefeller dissidents. A professor of economics and a professor of literature distinguished themselves by proclaiming that Rockefeller was "superior in creative genius to Shakespeare, Homer, and Dante". By comparison, another teacher, a Professor Bemis was expelled from the school for "incompetence" when he repeatedly criticized the action of the railroads during the Pullman strike of 1894. A few years later, after the Rockefeller family, through the "philanthropy" of John Archbald, had gained parallel influence at Syracuse University at western New York, an economics instructor by name of John Cummons was dismissed by the Chancellor for similar reasons.

IN 1953, Representative B. Carroll Reece of Tennessee received the authority of Congress to establish a special committee to investigate power and influence of tax-exempt foundations. The committee never got very far off the ground due to **mounting political pressure from sources high within government** itself and, eventually Reece was forced to terminate the work. During its short period of existence, however, many interesting and highly revealing facts were brought to light. Norman Dodd, who was the committee's director of research, and probably of the country's most knowledgeable authorities on foundations, testified during the hearings and told the committee: "**The result of the development and operation of the network in which the foundations (by their support and encouragement) have played such a significant role, seems to have provided this country with ... what is tantamount to a national system of education under the tight control of organizations and persons little known to the American public. . . . The curriculum in this tightly controlled scheme of education is designed to indoctrinate the American student from matriculation, to the consummation of his education.** (As quoted by Weaver, U.S. Philanthropic Foundation, op. cit., pp. 175, 176)".

UNDER THE CAREFUL supervision of Fred Gates, John D. Rockefeller set out consciously and methodically to capture control of American education and particularly of American medical education. The process began in **1901** with the creation of the **Rockefeller Institute for Medical Research**. It included on its board such politically oriented medical names as Doctor L. Emmett Holt, Christian A. Herter, T. Mitchell Pruden, Hermann M. Briggs, William H. Welch, Theobald Smith. and **Simon Flexner**. Christian Herter was slated for bigger things, of course, and became the secretary of State under President Eisenhower. Simon Flexner also was destined for larger success. Although his name never became as well-known as that of Herter, he and his brother, **Abraham Flexner**, probably **influenced the lives of more people** and in a more profound way than has any Secretary of State. Abraham Flexner was on the staff of the **Carnegie Foundation for the Advancement of Teaching**. As mentioned previously, the Rockefeller and Carnegie foundations traditionally worked together almost as one in the furtherance of their mutual goals, and this certainly was no exception. The Flexner brothers represented the lens that brought both the Rockefeller and the Carnegie fortunes into sharp focus on the unsuspecting and thoroughly vulnerable medical profession. Prior to 1910 the practice of medicine in the United States left a great deal to be desired. Some medical degrees could be purchased through the mail and many others could be obtained with marginal training at understaffed and inadequate medical schools. The profession was suffering from a bad public reputation and reform was in the air. The American Medical Association had begun to take an interest in cleaning its own house. It created a Council on Medical Education for the express purpose of surveying the status of medical training throughout the country and of making specific recommendations for its improvement. But by 1908 it had run into serious difficulty as a result of committee differences and insufficient funding. It was into this void that the Rockefeller-Carnegie combine moved with brilliant strategy and perfect timing. Henry S. Pritchett, the president of the Carnegie Foundation, approached the AMA (Author: AMA = The American Medical Association – the control body of the medical industry in the USA. Every country has such a control body.) and simply offered to take over the entire project. The minutes for the meeting of the AMA's Council on Medical Education held in New York in December of 1908 tell the story..,

AT ONE O' clock an informal conference was held with President Pritchett and Mr.Abraham Flexner of the Carnegie Foundation. Mr. Pritchett had already expressed by correspondence the willingness of the Foundation to cooperate with the Council in investigating the medical schools. He now explained that the **Foundation was to investigate all the professions: law, medicine, and, theology**.....

(1.THIS IS NOT the subject of the present study, but the reader should not pass over the fact that exactly the same strategy for control over education was being executed in other key areas as well. . .)

HE AGREED with the opinion previously expressed by the members of the Council that while the Foundation would be guided very largely by the Council's investigation - to avoid the usual claims of partiality, **no more mention should be made in the report of the Council than any other source of information**. The report would therefore be, and have the weight of a disinterested body, which would then be published far and wide. It would do much to develop public opinion.

[(2 'MORRIS FISHBEIN, M.D.A History of the AMA, (W.B. Saunders Co., Philadelphia & London. 1947). pp. 987, 989.]

"AND WHEN THEY **were assembled with the elders, and had taken counsel, they gave large money unto the soldiers**, Saying, Say ye, His disciples came by night, and stole him *away* while we slept. And if this come to the governor's ears, we will **persuade him, and secure you**. So **they took the money, and did as they were taught**: and this saying is commonly reported among the Jews **until this day**." (Matthew 28:12-15. (KJV)).

(AUTHOR: The rank and file, to this day, has not changed. Their allegiance can be bought. It also demonstrates the seduction of advertising – by paying large sums to the media, the media will say anything which the paymaster dictates. Remember Satan and his forces have <u>unlimited money</u> at their disposal).

HERE WAS the classical philanthropic formula at work again. Have others pay a major portion of the bill (the AMA had already done most of the work - (The total Carnegie investment was only $10 000), reap a large bonus from public opinion (isn't it wonderful that these men are taking an interest in upgrading medical education!), and gain an opportunity to control a large and vital sphere of American life. This is how that control came about.

THE **FLEXNER REPORT**, as it was called, was published in 1910. As anticipated, it was published far and wide, and it did do much to develop public opinion. The report quite correctly pointed out the inadequacies of medical education at the time. No one could take exception with that. It also proposed a wide range of sweeping changes, most of which were entirely sound. No one could take exception with those either. The alert researcher will note, however the recommendations **emphatically included the strengthening of courses in pharmacology and the addition of research departments at all "qualified" medical schools.**

(AUTHOR: Observe how cunning the strategy is! The complete strategy is reflected in one sentence namely: shift the focus away from natural healing to pharmaceuticals; create "research" which is censored according to the "scientific" model; failing which, the payer closes the purse strings of the university)

AND SO, the Flexner Report was above reproach and undoubtedly, it performed a service that was much needed at the time. It is what followed in the wake of the report that **reveals its true purpose in the total plan**. Rockefeller and Carnegie began immediately to shower **hundreds of millions of dollars on those better medical schools that were vulnerable to control.** Those that did not conform were denied the funds and the prestige that came with those funds - and were forced out of business.

A HUNDRED AND sixty medical schools were in operation in 1905. By 1927, the number had dropped to eighty. True, most of those that were edged out had been sub-standard. But so were some of those that received foundation money and survived. **The primary test was not their previous standing but their willingness to accept foundation influence and control.** Historian Joseph Goulden describes the process this way: Flexner had the idea, Rockefeller and Carnegie had the money, and their marriage was spectacular. The Rockefeller Institute for Medical Research and the General Education Board **showered money on tolerably respectable schools and on professors who expressed an interest in research.**

(1 Goulden. The Money Changers, op. Cit. p.141.)

SINCE 1910 THE foundations have invested over a billion dollars in the medical schools of America. **Nearly half of the faculty members now receive a portion of their income from foundation research grants and over sixteen percent of them are entirely funded this way. (Author: this is the visible tip of the iceberg).** Rockefeller and Carnegie have not been the only source of these funds. Substantial influence also has been exerted by the Ford Foundation, the Kellogg Foundation, the Commonwealth Fund (a Rockefeller interlock created by Edward Harkness of Standard Oil), the Sloan Foundation and the Macy Foundation.

THE FORD FOUNDATION has been extremely active in the field of medical education in recent years, but none of them can compare to the Rockefellers and the Carnegies for sheer money volume and historical continuity. Joseph C. Hinsey, in his highly authoritative paper entitled "The Role of Private Foundations in the Development of Modern Medicine", reviews the sequence of this expanding influence:

STARTING with Johns Hopkins Medical School in 1913, the General Education Board supported reorganizations which brought about full-time instruction in the **clinical as well as the basic science** departments for the first two years of medical education at Washington University in St. Louis, at Yale and at Chicago. In 1923, a grant was made to the University of Iowa in the amount of $2,250,000 by the General Education Board and the Rockefeller Foundation. Similar grants in smaller amounts were made to the following state supported medical schools: University of Colorado, University of Oregon, University of Virginia, and University of Georgia. An appropriation was made to the University of Cincinnati, an institution which received some of its support from municipal sources. Howard University and the Meharry Medical School were strengthened, the latter by some eight million dollars. The General Education Board and the Rockefeller Foundation later made substantial grants to the medical schools at Harvard, Vanderbilt, Columbia, Cornell, Tulane, Western Reserve, Rochester, Duke, Emory, and the Memorial Hospital in New York affiliated with Cornell.

THIS LIST, of course is not complete. It is necessary to add to it the medical schools of Northwestern, Kansas, and Rochester; each heavily endowed, either by Rockefeller money, or by the Commonwealth Fund which is closely aligned with Rockefeller interests.

AFTER ABRAHAM FLEXNER completed his report, he became one of the three most influential men in American medicine. The other two were, his brother, Dr. Simon Flexner of the Rockefeller Institute and Dr. William Welch of Johns Hopkins Medical School and of the Rockefeller Institute. According to Minsey, these men, acting as "**a triumvirate**":

(Author: Isn't this just something? Satan loves copying, in this case the Trinity)

... were not only involved in the awarding of grants for the Rockefeller Foundation, but they were **counselors to heads of institutions, to lay board members, to members of staffs of medical schools and universities in the United States and abroad**. They served as sounding boards, as stimulators of ideas and programs, as mediators in situations of difficulty.

THE ASSOCIATION of American Medical College has been one of the principal vehicles of foundation and cartel control over medical education in

DEMONISED DOCTORING

the United States and Canada. First organized in 1876 it served the function of setting a **wide range of standards** for all medical schools. It determines the criteria for selecting medical students, for curriculum development, for programs of continuing medical education after graduation, and for communication within the profession as well as to the general public. The Association of American Medical Colleges from its inception has been funded and dominated by the Commonwealth Fund, the China Medical Board (created in 1914 as a division or the Rockefeller Foundation), the Kellogg Foundation, the Macy, Markle, Rockefeller and Sloan foundations.

BY WAY OF ANALOGY, we may say that the **foundations captured control of the apex of the pyramid of medical education when they were able to place their own people onto the boards of the various schools and into key administrative positions.** The middle of the pyramid was secured by the Association of American Medical Colleges which set standards and unified the curricula. The base of the pyramid, however, was not consolidated until finally they were able to **select the teachers themselves**. Consequently, a major portion of foundation activity has always been directed toward what is generally called "**academic medicine**". Since 1913, the foundations have completely pre-empted this field. The Commonwealth Fund reports a half a million dollars in one year alone appropriated for this purpose, while the Rockefeller Foundation boasts of over **twenty thousand fellowships and scholarships** for the training of medical instructors.

IN THE MONEY GIVERS, Joseph Goulden touches upon this sensitive nerve when he says: "If the foundations chose to speak, their voice would resound with the solid clang of the **cash register**. Their expenditures on health and hospitals totaled more than a half-billion dollars between 1964 and a half 1968, according to a compilation by the American Association of Fund-Raising Counsel. But the foundations' "**innovative money**" goes for research, not for the production or doctors who treat human beings. **Medical schools, realizing this, paint their faces with the hue desired by their customers**".

Echoing this same refrain, David Hopgood writing in the Washington Monthly, says:

"The medical school curriculum and its entrance requirements are geared to the highly academic student who is headed for research. In the increasingly desperate struggle for admission, these **academically talented students are crowding out those who want to practice medicine**".

And so it has come to pass that the teaching staffs of all our medical schools are a very special breed. In the selection and training process, heavy emphasis always has been put on finding individuals who, because of temperament or special interest, have been attracted by the field of research, and especially by research in **pharmacology**. This has resulted in loading the staffs of our medical schools with men and women who, by preference and by training are ideal **propagators of the drug-oriented science** that has come to dominate American medicine. And the irony of it is that neither they nor their students are even remotely aware that they are products **of a rigid selection process geared to hidden commercial objectives**. So thorough is their insulation from this fact that **even when exposed to the obvious truth, very few are capable of accepting it**, for to do so would be a tremendous blow to their **professional pride**. Generally speaking, the deeper one is drawn into the medical profession, the more years he has been exposed to its regiments, the more difficult it is to break out of its confines. In practical terms this simply means that your doctor probably will be the last person on your Christmas card list to accept the facts presented in this study!

Dr. David L. Edsall at one time was the Dean of the Harvard Medical School. The conditions he describes at Harvard are the same as those at every other medical school in America: (and all first world universities; author).

"I was, for a period, a professor of therapeutics and pharmacology, and I knew from experience that students were obliged then by me and by others to learn about the interminable number of drugs, ... many of which were valueless, many of them useless, some probably even harmful .... Almost all subjects must be taken at exactly the same time, and in almost exactly the same way by all students, and the amount introduced into each course is such that few students have time or energy to explore any subject in a spirit of independent interest. A little comparison shows that there is less intellectual freedom in the medical course than in almost any other form of professional education in this country."

(L As quoted by Morris A. Bealle, The New Drug Story, (Columbia Publishing Co., Wash. D.C.. 1958). pp. 19. 20).

Yes, **he who pays the piper does call the tune**. It may not be humanly possible for those who finance the medical schools to determine what is taught in every minute detail. But such is not necessary to achieve the cartel's desired goals. One can be sure, however, that there is total control over what is not taught, and that, **under no circumstances will even one of Rockefeller's shiny dimes ever go to a medical college, to a hospital, to a teaching staff, or to a researcher that holds the unorthodox view that the best medicine is in nature.**

Because of its generous patron, **orthodoxy always will fiddle a tune of man-made drugs**. Whatever basic nutrition may be allowed into the melody will be minimal at best, and it will be played over and over again that natural sources of vitamins are in no way superior to those that are man-made or synthesized. **The day when orthodox medicine really embraces the field of nutrition will be the day when the cartel behind it also has monopolized the vitamin and food product industry essential to it** - not one day before.

(author: already in the making; the pharmaceutical/ medical/ industrial complex is currently involved in monopolizing all natural products – see chapter 9).

In the meantime, while doctors are forced to spend hundreds of hours studying the names and actions or all kinds of man-made drugs, they are lucky if they receive even a portion or a single course on basic nutrition. Many have none at all. The result is that the average doctor's wife or secretary knows more about practical nutrition than he does.

Returning to the main theme, however, we find that the cartel's influence over the field of orthodox medicine is felt far beyond the medical schools. After the doctor has struggled his way through ten or twelve years of learning what the cartels have decided is best for him to learn, he **then goes out into the world of medical practice and immediately is embraced by the other arm of cartel control - The American Medical Association.**

The global implementation of this strategy was easy because it simply became a "cooky cutter" exercise, meaning that the same recipe was then replicated throughout the western world. Pharmaceutical interests were firmly entrenched on a multinational scale, with the heart of the pharmaceutical industry being in Germany.

The pharmaceutical giant IG Farben had tentacles all over Europe.[9] It was also involved with the Rockefeller industries and Rothchild's. It also sponsored the nazi party during the second world war. It also has more than 200 000 trade agreements with allied interests in and around the world. Can the reader get the bigger picture of the morals that drove these interests?

It also had shares in the pharmaceutical/medical/industrial complex of America. The company, after the Nuremberg trials, is today better known as BASF, Bayer and Hoechst.

Taking some of the highlights from the above, the following aspects can be illustrated: "monopolized the vitamin and food product industry".

The pharmaceutical/medical/industrial complex is already implementing schemes which will render food, herbs, minerals and vitamins classified as drugs so that it can be prescribed at massive prices by doctors. See chapter 6.

"ORTHODOXY ALWAYS WILL FIDDLE a tune of man-made drugs".

THEY CANNOT STAND God's products.

"LEARN about the interminable number of drugs".

OVERWHELM (BRAINWASH) them with the diabolical information.

"GEARED TO HIDDEN COMMERCIAL OBJECTIVES".
   Occultic secret agendas.

"PHARMACOLOGY".

SORCERY, FROM THE GREEK "PHARMAKOS". Man made chemicals.

TO SUMMARIZE THIS CHAPTER, the pharmaceutical/medical/industrial complex has all the characteristics of a devilish plot. The doctor who has been trained and brainwashed by this system cannot but be demonised, and WILL believe the LIE.

EVEN IF HE (the doctor) claims to be a believer, he or she has been BLINDED in the field of healing. Perhaps the other areas of the demonised doctor's life are seemingly in order such as finances and family. If this book does not open the eyes of the demonised doctor, in spite of the Scriptural warnings and revelations provided in this and other books, then one is dealing with a certain manifestation which no book will solve, perhaps only by deliverance by the grace of God?

By establishing a dogma which could not be challenged, the medical industry had created one of the first cornerstones of a cult:

"**that the followers must accept without question whatever the cult leader (professor or teacher per the medical industry oath: inserted by author) as the infallible authority decrees**".

One of the most devastating statistics, indicating the rotten knowledge of health possessed by doctors, is their low life expectancy in the USA. In his audio tape entitled "Dead doctors don't lie", Dr. Wallach states that doctors have a life expectancy of 58 years, versus the years for other people. Very telling indeed!

References
1. Ephesians 6:11. (KJV).
2. Jeremiah 17:9-10. (KJV).
3. Kushi, Michio. *Natural healing through macrobiotics. Page 8. (1978)*
4. Hunt, Dave. *A woman rides the beast. (1994).*
5. Griffen, G. Edward. *World without cancer. (1978).*
6. Griffen, G. Edward. *World without cancer. Page 369-382 (1978).*
7. Matthew 28:12-15. (KJV).
8. 2 Thessalonians 2:11-12. (KJV).
9. Moss, Dr. Ralph W. *The cancer industry. Page 392. (1996)*
10. McAlvany, Donald S. *The McAlvany Intelligence Advisor. Page 17. November 1997.*
11. Hunt, Dave. *Occult Invasion. (1998).*

CHAPTER 5
WHAT IS SCIENCE?

One may ask the question: Goodbye God? Or Where is science? Is there a place for God and His creation in modern day science?

"But if our gospel be hid, it is hid to them that are lost: In whom the god of this world hath blinded the minds of them which believe not, lest the light of the glorious gospel of Christ, who is the image of God, should shine unto them. For we preach not ourselves, but Christ Jesus the Lord; and ourselves your servants for Jesus' sake."
 (2 Corinthians 4:3-5)

The unbeliever has been blinded by the devil, known as the "god of this world".

"For such are false apostles, deceitful workers, transforming themselves into the apostles of Christ. And no marvel; for Satan himself is transformed into an angel of light." (2 Corinthians 11:13-14. (KJV)).

SATAN APPEARS as a type of white knight saviour.

"THE SOWER SOWETH THE WORD. And these are they by the way side, where the word is sown; but when they have heard, Satan cometh immediately, and taketh away the word that was sown in their hearts." (Mark 4:14-15. (KJV)).

THE UNBELIEVER ("BY THE WAY SIDE") can hear the truth, but nevertheless, it will be "snatched away from them "immediately".

"FOR THERE SHALL ARISE false Christs, and false prophets, and shall shew great signs and wonders; insomuch that, if it were possible, they shall deceive the very elect." (Matthew 24:24. (KJV)).

THE "WONDERS" of modern science are so impressive that even the "very elect" of the true believers would be in danger of being deceived.

FOR THE INVISIBLE things of him from the creation of the world are clearly seen, being understood by the things that are made, even his eternal power and Godhead; so that they are without excuse: Because that, when they knew God, they glorified him not as God, neither were thankful; but became vain in their imaginations, and their foolish heart was darkened. (Romans 1:21. (KJV)).

GOD REVEALS EVEN some invisible mysteries of His creation to humans (including unbelievers). Instead of accepting these mysterious revelations and crediting God, humans "invent" their own stupid explanations for these phenomena.

"THROUGH FAITH we understand that the worlds were framed by the word

of God, so that things which are seen were not made of things which do appear." (Hebrews 11:3. (KJV)).

SCIENTISTS HAVE a huge problem with this principle. The universe or "worlds" were created by the "word" (word = sound = energy), so that visible matter ("things") actually consist of immaterial things (something which is not a particle). Psychics and real healers have known this all along. Unfortunately the believers have been deceived away from this avenue of truth by the seductive "imaginings" of scientists. The unbelievers on the other hand, who have utilized the energies of God's creation, have given credit to their false gods for this power. A brilliant strategy by the "father of the lie"! The result is that the believers don't get the benefit of free Godly energetics, and the unbelievers use it to further promote occultic beliefs. This Godly energy is abused particularly viciously in the attacks by upholders of the "scientific religion". They employ the arguments to scare believers away from natural healing by labeling the word "energy" as "occultic". Just another diabolical deception to herd gullible believers back to the pharmaceutical/medical/industrial torture chamber.

"BUT EVIL MEN and seducers shall wax worse and worse, deceiving, and being deceived." (2 Timothy 3:13 (KJV)).

THE DECEIVERS ARE subject to the same deception which they themselves are perpetrating.

"WHILE WE LOOK NOT at the things which are seen, but at the things which are not seen: for the things which are seen are temporal; but the things which are not seen are eternal." (2 Corinthians 4:18. (KJV)).

THE MATERIAL or visible world is not as important as the invisible world, in an eternal context.

Ever learning, and never able to come to the knowledge of the truth. (2 Timothy 3:7 (KJV)).

Because the truth is not in learning, but in gaining wisdom and understanding God's word. This is a sobering concept for all the professors, including the theologians.

And ye shall <u>know</u> the truth, and the truth shall make you free.

Jesus said <u>knowing</u> the truth shall set you free, and <u>not</u> the truth shall set you free.

One of the most knowledgeable students of the New World Order process, Dave Icke, missed this point when he titled his exposé book "And the truth shall set you free". (The back cover of his book does however use the correct context).

The lesson is that unbelievers should not quote from the Bible since they might use the quote out of context and be identified with Satan, because using the Bible out of context is the signature of Satan.

In this chapter the reader will learn that major components of science is a massive lie and fraud on the world. It is so subtle and pervasive that even the "elect" are in danger of being deceived. As far as the author of this book is aware, only a few authors from the Christian community are in print as having partially recognized this scientific deception. Four of them are Dave Hunt, Donald S McAlvaney, Clifford Oden and Walter Veith. The others authors seem to have been "taken", hook, line and sinker by the "scientific religion".

MOST OF THE Christian believers have, like a pack of baying hounds, followed the popular trendy chorus line of "alternative medicine is occultic". Little do they realize that this was simply a brilliant plan, hatched by the pharmaceutical/medical/ industrial complex and their CEO (chief executive officer), Satan, to deceive humans. As a red herring, it is masterful! By using the genuine occultic component of the natural healing industry, as the big lie, to lump all the "opposition" under the same blanket classification, the medical goal had been attained. Western scientific medicine has been vindicated as the ultimate scientific, non-occultic magic road to eternal health! The health saviour had arrived. And so, the best lies are always cloaked in partial truth!

BELIEVERS, and the others, were now assured of spiritual safety when seeking healing. All they had to do was abdicate their health to a medical industry professional! Your doctor knows best! Consult your doctor! If in doubt, consult a doctor! If it stings, won't go away, is red, is black, is strange, is sore, is dull, is pregnant, is unusual, is anything, then see your doctor. (The doctor would be sure to save you from eternal illness, and find something to test and treat). The relentless propaganda mill of the pharmaceutical/medical/industrial complex has churned out movies, TV programs, commercials and health articles, all to the same effect.

NORMAL LIFE PROCESSES have now become "treatable diseases". So from conception, pregnancy, puberty, menopause and senility, all stages of life have become "diseases" which can only be assessed by a doctor. He can then perform continuous tests and treatments on people with the "latest" "break-through" technology. Some how or other, the "latest" "break-through" technology is always improved upon, rendering the previous "latest" "break-through" technology obsolete. How can the one "ultimate" status be replaced by another "ultimate" status? That is exactly how clothing fashions are perpetuated.

THE COMMON "COOKIE CUTTER" or mass produced doctor only has vague suspicions that something is amiss. While his social and financial status is assured by the pharmaceutical/medical/industrial complex, he has no incentive to "rock the boat" or improve matters, since it could jeopardize his cosy comfort zone of social status and good income. This comfort zone is arranged for him by the powers who know human frailties all to well, namely, the Satan contrived and controlled pharmaceutical/medical/industrial complex.

ONE CAN IMAGINE what the Scriptural view on this deception would be. Humans may make many claims as to their abilities, for instance toastmasters, carpenters, insurance brokers, pilots, and many more. However, according to Scripture, for one to make a claim as a "healer", one needs Scriptural grounds to claim it .

"IN THAT DAY **shall he swear, saying, I will not be an <u>healer</u>; for in my house is neither bread nor clothing: make me not a ruler of the people.**" (Isaiah 3:7. (KJV)).

HAVE ALL the <u>gifts of healing</u>? (1 Corinthians 12:30. (KJV)).

"TO ANOTHER FAITH **by the same Spirit; to another the <u>gifts of healing</u> by the same <u>Spirit</u>.**" (1 Corinthians 12:9 (KJV)).

HOW GOD ANOINTED Jesus of Nazareth with the Holy Ghost and with power: who went about doing good, and <u>healing all that were oppressed of the devil.</u> (Acts 10:38 (KJV)).

"AND THEY DEPARTED, **and went through the towns, preaching the gospel, and <u>healing</u> every where.**" (Luke 9:6 (KJV)).

"AND GOD HATH **set some in the church, first apostles, secondarily prophets, thirdly teachers, after that miracles, then <u>gifts of healing</u>, helps, governments, diversities of tongues.**" (1 Corinthians 12:28. (KJV)).

"**Is any sick among you? let him call for the elders of the church; and let them pray over him, anointing him with oil in the name of the Lord: And the prayer of faith shall <u>save the sick</u>...**" (James 5:14-15 (KJV)).

FROM THE ABOVE verses of Scripture it would seem that, to be a healer, one does not need the sanction of a Rockefeller approved, scientific, state sponsored, medically approved, board sanctioned, licensed, degreed, paid up, peer reviewed, socially accepted, and Satan liked, double blind placebo controlled tested qualification to heal a sick and/or suffering fellow human being. According to Scripture all you need is a <u>gift</u> from God, or an appointment in the church, or be an elder. But that would be "unscientific"! Anyone making healing claims is breaking the law in first world countries, and will be arrested and curtailed. Only doctor's are permitted to make healing claims!

GOD'S WAY is NOT scientific. Science is humanity's pathetic attempt at trying to describe the visible parts of God's creation, and then perverting it to suit their own agenda of the moment. Since the major component of the creation is invisible, the "brilliant scientists" will never get to the truth if they elect to keep God out of the equation. The only way they will ever know the truth about nature, will be when God chooses to reveal it to them.

YE ARE of <u>your father the devil</u>, and the lusts of your father ye will do. He was a murderer from the beginning, and <u>abode not in the truth</u>, because there is no truth in him. When he speaketh a lie, he speaketh of his own: for <u>he is a liar, and the father of it</u>. (John 8:44. (KJV)).

STRONG WORDS from Jesus Christ Himself! He says that the unbeliever is a child of the devil, and that the devil is the father of the lie.

PERHAPS THE DEFINITION of what science is supposed to mean, would help the reader to clear the clutter which has been created by the "spin doctors" (propaganda specialists) during a lifetime of deceptive education. By this implication is meant that there exists real science as well as fake science or "scientific religion".

FROM A DICTIONARY PERSPECTIVE, the definition of science reads:

SCIENCE (NOUN):
1. Systematic study and <u>knowledge</u> of natural or physical phenomena.
2. Any branch of study concerned with <u>observed material</u> facts.

THE REAL SCIENCE deals with <u>facts</u>. (An idea, religion, theory, dogma, hypothesis or political position is not a fact).

DIFFERENCES BETWEEN "REAL" SCIENCE AND FAKE "SCIENCE"

REAL SCIENCE vs FAKE SCIENCE
  1. Upholds creationism.
  Upholds evolution theory and natural selection.
  2. Studies all of God's creation, including His Word.
  Studies only what is selected by the dictates of superiors.
  3. Cannot be easily corrupted.
  Is easily corrupted.
  4. Goal is knowledge.
  Goal is not obvious. (profit)
  5. Used for technological progress.
  Used for hidden, private advantage.
  6. Based on Godly principles.
  Based on human principles.
  7. Unproven theories are dropped.
  Clings to unproven theories.
  8. Not intended for evil purposes.
  Intended for evil (or money) agenda.
  9. Rejected if error is proven.

Errors not necessarily rejected.
10. Defended mildly.
Violently defended.
11. Principles are simple.
Convoluted principles.
12. Energy effective.
Energy ineffective.
13. Does not damage nature.
Damaging to nature.
14. Considers long term effect.
Short term view is paramount.
15. Tolerant of criticism.
Intolerant to criticism.
16. Encourages innovation.
Intolerant to innovation.
17. Freedom of expression.
Severe censorship.
18. No suppression of new discoveries.
Competing discoveries suppressed.
19. Is open to public scrutiny.
Secretive.
20. Has automatic safeguards.
Has unpleasant side-effects.

ONE OF THE most devastating dogmas entrenched by the medical "scientific religion" is the "double blind, placebo controlled, crossover study". It has become the "gold standard" of the medical industry, (meaning that the person who has the gold will set the standards).

WHAT THIS CONVOLUTED method secretly intended, was equivalent to the Inquisition by the church in the middle ages. The authorities would haul anyone who disagreed with them, before the Inquisition. If this person chose to deviate from the dogma, it was called "anathema" (cursed), and they would be drastically punished. Thus there was only one way, and that was the way of the church. The pharmaceutical/medical/ industrial complex has invented the modern version of the Inquisition, namely the "double blind, placebo controlled, crossover study". What it actually is, is a "double-cross, blinded, placebo concocted" study. The underlying rationale for this abomination is that:

THE SCIENTISTS MUST NOT KNOW which is the test group and which is the control group, hence "double blind". So the observer is left in the dark. Occultic means unknown", remember. The participants do not know what is going on!

"PLACEBO CONTROLLED" means the effect on the experiment, of the mind of the observers, as well as the effect of the minds of the test subjects (patients), must be eliminated. This is a tautology, (dog chasing-it's-own-tail-argument), since the effect of the mind on healing has been measured as high as 30% of the healing effect. When a medicine is tested the placebo effect should therefore be INCLUDED! By eliminating it, the true value of the medicine will never be known.

"CROSSOVER" means that about halfway through the experiment, the whole exercise has to be switched around so that only the "statistically significant" results show up. In other words the control group now becomes the group receiving the active substance.

Any healing modality which does not "pass" this test is dismissed as "unscientific". The hurdles have been designed by Satan to cause untold confusion, and specifically to exclude human observation and the power of belief out of the conclusions.

"DESPISE NOT PROPHESYING. **Prove all things; hold fast that which is good. Abstain from all appearance of evil.**" (1 Thessalonians 5:20-22 (KJV)).

HOW DOES ONE "PROVE ALL THINGS"? Not by "double blind, placebo controlled, crossover study"! One proves it by Scripture , or by empirical tests (experience), or by observation or anecdote (telling someone about it).

THE "DOUBLE BLIND, placebo controlled, crossover study" has been specifically designed to exclude experience and Scripture. The worst accusation (anathema), that the pharmaceutical/medical/industrial complex can level at natural healing is that it is "anecdotal"(a very short story dealing with an incident). Since the anecdote does not comply with the "double blind, placebo controlled, crossover study", it is rejected by "scientific religion". The whole sinister goal of the "scientific religion" is to develop standards which exclude the Bible and God's methods from being accepted as evidence. All of the Bible is "ANECDOTAL" because the main theme is the "STORY OF THE CROSS". No one can prove God, Christ or the Holy Spirit with the "double blind, placebo controlled, crossover study". That is the way it was designed.

ANOTHER CRITIC OF THE "SCIENTIFIC RELIGION" sees it this way:

IN CASE the difference between evidence and medical evidence or the difference between facts and scientific facts elude you, let me explain. If I have a headache or a fever, that's not a fact except to me. If I tell a doctor about it, that's what doctors call anecdotal evidence or testimonial. If the doctor takes my temperature and writes it down, the headache becomes medical evidence. If another doctor copies it, it becomes a scientific fact. Should I need proof that my fever was 101 last Tuesday and ask my doctor for my chart, it will not be given to me. That plain garden variety fact has now become a scientific fact. It's only available to another doctor. If I complain that the doctor won't give me the scientific facts about my past condition, that's anecdotal evidence again.

WHEN TESTING EXTREMELY TOXIC DRUGS, the "double blind, placebo controlled, crossover study" has merits. Even so, thousands of drugs which "passed" the tests, have subsequently been withdrawn from the market because of poor performance and/or toxicity which were not revealed by the test. The conclusion one can draw from this is that the "double blind, placebo controlled, crossover study" is not very effective at revealing dangers, but highly effective at keeping natural medicines out of the market.

Most of the natural healing mechanisms designed by God will also fail this double blind etc. test, because it was designed to make only the man-made mechanisms look good.

There are of course degrees, or a mixture of both sides of good and bad science in certain industries, since all secular organizations are Godless. The pharmaceutical/ medical/industrial complex is, however engaged in a special mission of Satan, and not merely Godless.

The author is not suggesting that there should not be standards. The objection raised here is that standards should be fair, appropriate and correctly applied. Randomized controlled trials are valuable tools in research. However, by eliminating the placebo component, the whole purpose is defeated since the placebo phenomenon is an integral component of healing.

The manner in which the pharmaceutical/medical/industrial complex tortures the statistics, is what the author is objecting to.

A question which frequently puzzles naïve students, is the issue of orchestration. They cannot believe that someone, somewhere, has planned the status quo. It takes a giant paradigm shift for an unbeliever to realize that there are "principalities and powers" who orchestrate world affairs in preparation for centralized control. Scholars of the Scriptures, if they are believers, have no difficulty in grasping the idea of global manipulation since it is a major theme of end time prophesy. One of the most enthusiastic authors on this subject is Texe Marrs. An excerpt from one of his book covers provides a succinct overview:
    (Emphasis and bracketed comments by author).

Is man on the very threshold of becoming a god? New Age teachers say we are soon to enter a marvelous new era of peace, prosperity and superhuman status. On the horizon are incredible **scientific achievements**: lifelike robots to become our companions, **miracle drugs** to blot out guilt and provide sexual ecstasy (Author: Viagra), and fantastic computer biochips that can be surgically inserted into our brains to give us genius-level intelligence. Texe Marrs, in MEGA FORCES, points to a shocking and chilling truth: behind the shiny facade of New Age teachings and **scientific progress** lies Satan's blueprint for chaos and destruction. The world is being prepared economically and politically for a despicable era of unbelief, turmoil and persecution. **Science is inventing horrible new weapons of war** and producing advanced torture tools which the coming **Antichrist will readily use to control and ravage**. The spectre of tribulation, holocaust, and Armageddon loom large in man's bitter future. **All this is prophesied in our Holy Bible**. It will come to pass, perhaps far sooner than you might think.

EVEN THE UNBELIEVERS can read the signs. There is a catch though; the New Agers believe that the end times will herald improvements. The Bible states that the end times will herald the worst tribulation that the world has ever known. This subject is outside the scope of this book, but needs to be known in order to illustrate the prime role of western medicine and the pharmaceutical/medical/industrial complex in the devastation of human freedom.

ANOTHER DIFFICULT CONCEPT for deceived people to grasp is the fact that "all the people can get fooled all the time" by this grand scientific fraud. They cannot comprehend why the fraud was not stopped or disclosed. To understand it one needs to merge two ideas, namely, the gullibility of humans and the craftiness of the architects of the scheme. Human error or frailty is only one side of the transaction. The other side is the sinister and powerful groups who plan and maintain it all.

ABOUT THREE HUNDRED years ago the master plan to corrupt science was hatched. Without this plan the pharmaceutical/medical/industrial complex would be unable to destroy freedom of health on the earth.

The history was well studied by a secular scientist and ardent critic of his own scientific world. Being a critic, he was of course ostracized. Here are excerpts from his one book, "The turning Point", by Dr. Fritjof Capra:

(Emphasis and bracketed comments by author)

THE WORLD VIEW and value system that lie at the basis of our culture and that have to be carefully reexamined were formulated in their essential outlines in the sixteenth and seventeenth centuries. **Between 1500 and 1700 there was a dramatic shift in the way people pictured the world** and in their whole way of thinking. The new mentality and the new perception of the cosmos gave our Western civilization the features that are characteristic of the modern era. They became the basis of the **paradigm that has dominated our culture for the past three hundred years** and is now about to change.

BEFORE 1500 THE dominant world view in Europe, as well as in most other civilizations, was organic. **People lived in small, cohesive communities and experienced nature in terms of organic relationships, characterized by the interdependence of spiritual and material phenomena and the subordination of individual needs to those of the community.** The scientific framework of this organic-world view rested on two authorities - **Aristotle and the Church. In the thirteenth century Thomas Aquinas combined Aristotle's comprehensive system of nature with Christian theology and ethics and, in doing so, established the conceptual framework that remained unquestioned throughout the Middle Ages.** The nature of medieval science was very different from that of contemporary science. It was based on both reason and faith and its main goal was to **understand the** meaning and **significance of things, rather than prediction and control. Medieval scientists, looking for the purposes underlying various natural phenomena, considered questions relating to God, the human soul, and ethics to be of the highest significance.**

THE MEDIEVAL OUTLOOK changed radically in the sixteenth and seventeenth centuries. The notion of an organic, living, and **spiritual universe was replaced by that of the world as a machine, and the world-machine** became the dominant metaphor of the modern era. This development was brought about by revolutionary changes in physics and astronomy, culminating in the achievements of **Copernicus, Galileo, and Newton**. The science of the seventeenth century was based on a new method of inquiry, **advocated forcefully by Francis Bacon**, which involved the mathematical description nature and the analytic method of reasoning conceived by the genius of Descartes. Acknowledging the crucial role of science in bringing about these far-reaching changes, historians have called the sixteenth and seventeenth centuries the Age of the Scientific Revolution.

THE SCIENTIFIC REVOLUTION began with Nicolas **Copernicus, who overthrew the geocentric view of Ptolmy and the Bible** that had been accepted dogma for more than a thousand years. After Copernicus, the earth was no longer the center of the universe but merely one of the many planets circling a minor star at the edge of the galaxy **robbing man of his proud position as the central figure of God's creation**. Copernicus was fully aware that his view would deeply offend the religious consciousness of his time; he delayed its publication until 1543, the year of his death, and even then he presented the heliocentric view merely as a hypothesis.

COPERNICUS WAS FOLLOWED by **Johannes Kepler**, a scientist and **mystic** who searched for the harmony of the spheres and was able, through painstaking work with astronomical tables, to formulate his celebrated empirical laws of planetary motion, which gave further support to the Copernican system. But the real change in scientific opinion was brought about by Galileo Galilei, who was already famous for discovering the law of falling bodies when he turned his attention to astronomy. Directing the newly invented telescope to the skies and applying his extraordinary gift for scientific observation to celestial phenomena, Galileo was able to discredit the old cosmology beyond any doubt and to establish the Copernican hypothesis as a valid scientific theory.

THE ROLE of Galileo in the Scientific Revolution goes far beyond his achievements in astronomy, although these are most widely known because of his

clash with the Church. Galileo was the first to combine scientific experimentation with the use of mathematical language to formulate the laws of nature, he discovered, and is therefore considered the father of modern science. Philosophy* he believed, "is written in that great book which ever lies before your eyes; but we cannot understand it if we do not first learn the language and characters in which it is written. This language is mathematics, and the characters are triangles, circles, and other geometric figures."

TWO ASPECTS of his empirical approach and his use of a mathematical description of nature, became the dominant features of science in the seventeenth century and have remained important criteria of scientific theories up to the present day.

TO MAKE **it possible for scientists to describe nature mathematically,** Galileo postulated that they **should restrict themselves to studying the essential properties of material bodies** – shapes, numbers and movement - which could be **measured and quantified.** Other properties, like color, sound, taste, or smell were merely subjective mental projections which should be excluded from the domain of science. Galileo's strategy of directing the scientist's attention to the quantifiable properties of matter has proved extremely successful throughout modern science, but it has also exacted a heavy toll. As the psychiatrist R. D. Laing emphatically reminds us: "**Out go sight, sound, taste, touch and smell and along with them has since gone aesthetics and ethical sensibility, values, quality, form; all feelings, motives, intentions, soul, consciousness, spirit.** Experience as such is cast out of the realm of scientific discourse." According to Laing **hardly anything has changed our world more during the past four hundred years than the obsession of scientists with measurement and quantification.**

WHILE GALILEO DEVISED ingenious experiments in Italy, **Francis Bacon** set forth the empirical method of science explicitly in **England.** Bacon was the first to formulate a clear theory of the inductive procedure - to make experiments and to draw general conclusions from them, to be tested in further experiments - and he became extremely influential by vigorously advocating the new method. **He boldly attacked traditional schools** of thought and developed a veritable passion for scientific experimentation.

...Since Bacon, the goal of science has been knowledge that can be used to dominate and control nature and today both science and the technology are used predominantly for purposes that are profoundly anti-ecological.

The terms in which Bacon advocated his new empirical method of investigation were not only passionate but often outright vicious. Nature, in his view had to be "hounded in her wanderings," "bound into service" and made a "slave".

She was to be "**put in constraint**", and the aim of the scientist was **to "torture nature's secrets from her"**. Much of this violent imagery seems to have been inspired by the witch trials which were held frequently in Bacon's time. As attorney general for King James 1, Bacon was intimately familiar with such prosecutions, and because nature was commonly seen as female, it is not surprising that he should carry over the metaphors used in the courtroom into his scientific writings. **Indeed, his view of nature as a female whose secrets have to be tortured from her with the help of mechanical devices is strongly suggestive of the widespread torture of women in witch trials** of the early seventeenth century. Bacon's work thus represents an outstanding example of the influence of patriarchal attitudes on scientific thought.

Scientific Revolution proceeded to replace the organic view of nature with the **metaphor of the world as a machine**. This shift, which was to become of overwhelming importance for the further development of Western civilization, was initiated and completed by two towering figures, **Descartes and Newton.**

René Descartes is usually regarded as the **founder of modern philosophy**. He was a brilliant mathematician and his philosophical outlook was profoundly affected by the new physics and astronomy. He did not accept any traditional knowledge, but set out to build a whole new system of thought. According to Bertrand Russell, "This had not happened since Aristotle, and is a sign of the new confidence that resulted from the progress of science. There is a freshness about his work that is not to be found in any eminent previous philosopher since Plato."

AT THE AGE OF TWENTY-THREE, Descartes experienced an illuminating vision that was to shape his entire life. After several hours of intense concentration, during which he reviewed systematically all the knowledge he had accumulated, he perceived, in a **sudden flash of intuition, the "foundations of a marvelous science" which promised the unification of all knowledge.** This intuition had been foreshadowed in a letter to a friend in which Descartes announced his ambitious aim: "And so as to not hide anything from you about the nature of my work, I would like to give the public . . . a completely new science which **would resolve generally all questions of quantity, continuous or discontinuous**". In his vision Descartes perceived how he could realize this plan. He saw a method that would allow him to construct a complete science of nature about which he could have absolute certainty; a science based, like mathematics, on self-evident first principles. Descartes was overwhelmed by his revelation. He felt that he had made the supreme discovery of his life and had no doubt that **his vision came from divine inspiration. (Author: This is how Satan works, as a "divine" deceiver)** This conviction was enforced by an extraordinary dream the following night in which the new science was presented to him in symbolic form. Descartes was now **certain that God had shown him** his mission and he set out to build a scientific philosophy.

DESCARTES' vision had implanted in him the firm belief in the certainty of scientific knowledge, and his vocation in life was to distinguish **truth** from error in all fields of learning, "All science is certain, evident knowledge", he wrote. "We reject all knowledge which is merely probable and judge that only those things should be believed which are perfectly known and about which there can be no doubts.

The belief in the certainty of scientific knowledge lies at the very basis of Cartesian philosophy and of the world view derived from it, and it is here at the very outset, that Descartes went wrong. Twentieth-century physics has shown us very forcefully that **there is no absolute truth in science**, that all our concepts and theories are limited and approximate. The Cartesian belief in scientific truth is still widespread today and is reflected in the scientism that has become typical of our Western culture. Many people in our society, scientists as well as **non-scientists, are convinced that the scientific method is the only valid way of understanding the universe**. Descartes' method of thought and his view of nature have influenced all branches of modern science...

By the way, Sir Francis Bacon was a Masonic master and Grand Commander of the Rosicrucians.

So the scene was set, in all of the western world, for the new paradigm of "I think, therefore I am" of Descartes (the famous slogan of his). All human values had been removed from science. God was out of the picture, so the next players could move in.

Next to enter the stage was Newton. Here is an historical account:

Before Newton there had been two opposing trends in seventeenth-century science; the empirical, inductive method represented by **Bacon** and the rational, deductive method represented by **Descartes**. Newton, in his Principia, introduced the **proper mixture of both methods**, emphasizing that neither experiments without systematic interpretation nor deduction from first principles without experimental evidence will lead to a reliable theory. Going beyond Bacon in his systematic experimentation and beyond Descartes in his mathematical analysis, Newton unified the two trends and developed a **methodology upon which natural science has been based ever since**.

Isaac Newton was a much more complex personality than one would think from a reading of his scientific writings. He excelled not only as a scientist and mathematician but also, at various stages of his life, as a lawyer, historian, and **theologian**, and he was **deeply involved in research into occult and esoteric knowledge**. He looked at the world as a riddle and believed that its clues could be found not only through scientific experiments but also in the **cryptic revelations of esoteric traditions. Newton was tempted to think, like Descartes, that his powerful mind could unravel all the secrets of the universe, and he applied it with equal intensity to the study of natural and esoteric science.** While working at Trinity College, Cambridge, on the Principia, he accumulated, during the very same years, **voluminous notes on alchemy, apocalyptic texts, unorthodox theological theories, and various occult matters**. Most of these esoteric writings have never been published, but what is known of them indicates that **Newton, the great genius of the Scientific Revolution, was at the same time the "last of the magicians."**

So the founding fathers of the "scientific religion" consisted of Descartes, the "I am"; Bacon the Masonic master; and Newton the "last of the magicians". No wonder they had, and have, the whole world fooled! By the way, by reading the following two verses one can see who Descartes was counterfeiting with his famous saying! Not satisfied with deceiving people, he appropriated God's title for himself.

"Jesus said unto them, **Verily, verily, I say unto you, Before Abraham was, I am.**" (John 8:58. (KJV)).

"And God said unto Moses, **I AM THAT I AM: and he said, Thus shalt thou say unto the children of Israel, I AM hath sent me unto you.**" (Exodus 3:14. (KJV)).

Next to enter the stage is a person who has turned the whole "scientific religion" into the laughing stock of the true believers, as well as a joke to the satanists (satanists at least know that God exists, whereas "scientific religion" does not). Enter Charles Darwin of the "chance mutation and natural selection" fame, or better known as the neo-Darwinist theory of synthetic evolution. For brevity, the term "simple evolution theory" will be used. There is ample evidence of evolutionary processes on earth. This evidence has however been tortured and perverted to conform to the idea that there is no creative God.

THIS IDEA, on which countless quantities of money, time and effort have been spent, by billions of people, can only be described as utmost trash, and hilarious as well! Even serious defenders of the "scientific religion", when they think carefully, are embarrassed by the ridiculous ideas of the simple evolution theory

THERE IS meticulous evidence by the author Ian Taylor in his book "In the Minds of Men : Darwin and the New World Order", of how Darwin was set up to "manufacture" the whole deception of the theory in order to control the minds of humans.

DOCTORS, and other students at medical schools are brainwashed with this evolution trash in their junior years. It does not take much more doing at university, since the junior and senior schools' curricula do the brainwashing for many years prior to university. To make sure the doctor understands the fact that humans were not created by God, they are taught, in anatomy class, about "vestigial" organs in humans. This is a name given to human organs, in cases where the "scientific religion" has not determined the function of the particular organ! These organs are then called "vestigial" which means: "latent", "rudimentary" or "undeveloped". This creates the impression that:
1. God made a mistake.
2. The organ is not yet fully "evolved" on it's journey which lead to humans becoming "gods".
3. It's a leftover from the "caveman stage" of evolution.

THIS TYPE of training explains the phenomenon whereby doctors readily butcher tonsils out of children, with very little idea that God planned a vital role for tonsils. The removal of other organs such as wombs, gall bladders, appendixes and prostate glands are just as easily carried out, leaving the doctor richer and the patient maimed and malfunctional for life.

THE DEVILISH CONCEPT of the "simple evolution theory" is promoted with fervor all over the western world. The author, in 1997, witnessed the brainwashing during a visit to the multi million pound British Museum of Natural History in London. Here, high-tech, glitzy, and very impressive displays reinforce the "evolution theory". Busloads of impressionable school children, and hordes of gullible tourists are mind-damaged there for life. One would be surprised to find out who the promoters and supporters of this abomination are. Yes, the pharmaceutical/medical/industrial complex! And the British taxpayer subsidizes it!

ANOTHER ISSUE of serious concern about the "scientific religion" community is the question: If the doctors can believe trash such as the "evolution theory", which other, more subtle falsehoods are not slipping through their academic "armor" of discernment?

AS FAR AS TECHNOLOGY GOES, technology based on "scientific religion" will always have hidden dangers built in, while technology based on "real science" will have built-in and honest safeguards, as well as useful improvements for humans. An example of "real" technology is the continuous improvements in saw blades and cutting tools. Compare this to the false technology of antibiotics which have got progressively more harmful and more useless, as time progressed.

AS THE READER can see by now, "scientific religion" not only rests on occultic foundations, but has spawned an even more perverted sub-division called medical "scientific religion". It is in the pagan temples, medical industry schools, where the cookie-cutter doctors (mass produced) are brainwashed, and then unleashed in a genocidal orgy on the world.

References
1. 2 Corinthians 4:3-5. (KJV).
2. 2 Corinthians 11:13-14. (KJV).
3. Mark 4:14-15. (KJV).
4. Matthew 24:24. (KJV).
5. Romans 1:21. (KJV).
6. Hebrews 11:3. (KJV).
7. 2 Timothy 3:13 (KJV).
8. 2 Corinthians 4:18. (KJV).
9. Hunt, Dave. *The seduction of Christianity. (1985).*
10. McAlvany, Donald S. *The McAlvany Intelligence Advisor. Page 17. November 1997.*
11. Oden, Rev. Clifford. *Thank God I have cancer. Page 90-92. (1976)*
12. Veith, Dr. Walter. *Diet and health, new scientific perspectives. (1993).*
13. Isaiah 3:7. (KJV).
14. 1 Corinthians 12:30. (KJV).
15. 1 Corinthians 12:9. (KJV).
16. Act 10:38. (KJV).
17. Luke 9:6. (KJV).
18. Icke, Dave. *And the truth shall set you free. (1997)*
19. **Collins compact dictionary of the English language.** *(1984)*
20. Marrs, Texe. *Mega Forces. (1989).*
21. Capra, Dr. Fritjof. *The turning point. p37-52 (1983).*
22. John 8:58. (KJV).
23. Exodus 3:14. (KJV).
24. Milton, Richard. *The facts of life. Shattering the myths of Darwinism. (1993)*
25. 1 Thessalonians 5:20-22. (KJV).
26. 1 Corinthians 12:28 (KJV).
27. James 5:14-15 (KJV).
28. Icke, Dave. *And the truth shall set you free. p33 (1997).*
29. Taylor, Ian T. *In the Minds of Men : Darwin and the New World Order.(1991).*
30. Dufty, William. *Sugar Blues. Page 93. (1975).*

CHAPTER 6
KNOW THE TREE BY IT'S FRUIT

"Now the works of the flesh are manifest, which are these; Adultery, fornication, <u>uncleanness</u>, lasciviousness, <u>Idolatry</u>, <u>witchcraft</u>, <u>hatred</u>, <u>variance</u>, <u>emulations</u>, <u>wrath</u>, <u>strife</u>, seditions, <u>heresies</u>, <u>envyings</u>, <u>murders</u>, drunkenness, revellings, and <u>such like</u>: of the which I tell you before, as I have also told you in time past, that they which do such things shall <u>not inherit the kingdom of God</u>." (Galatians 5:19-21)

"BUT THE FRUIT of the Spirit is love, joy, peace, longsuffering, gentleness, goodness, faith, meekness, temperance..." (Galations 5:22-23)

THE APOSTLE PAUL lists the results which the Holy Spirit brings forth in believers. It is not expected that the secular world would display these good fruits. This Scripture quotes the one extreme of the "fruit" spectrum. The accounting profession (the control group) would feature somewhere in the middle ground, where there is a mix of good fruit and bad fruit. The medical industry would feature on the other extreme, where the bulk of their fruit is not only bad, but outright evil.

"BEWARE OF FALSE PROPHETS, which come to you in sheep's clothing, but inwardly they are ravening wolves. Ye shall know them by their fruits. Do men gather grapes of thorns, or figs of thistles? Even so every good tree bringeth forth good fruit; but a corrupt tree bringeth forth evil fruit. A good tree cannot bring forth evil fruit, neither can a corrupt tree bring forth good fruit. Every tree that bringeth not forth good fruit is hewn down, and cast into the fire. Wherefore by their fruits ye shall know them." (Matthew 7:15-20. (KJV)).

JESUS CHRIST STATES the principle whereby the moral status of the tree might be identified. Note that He does not say that the tree is known by it's intentions, credo, history, wealth, knowledge, social status or other criteria – only by it's fruit.

THE PHARMACEUTICAL/MEDICAL/INDUSTRIAL complex deserves a special place in the ranks of evil "fruit trees" of this world. The extremely subtle deception is so diabolical that it could not possibly have originated in the limited human mind. Compared to, for instance the pornography industry, the medical industry is hidden behind many veils of and layers of deception and mystery. The pornography industry, although evil, is not difficult to identify – very little discernment is required to recognize what the industry practices. The medical industry, on the other hand, presents the façade of "health care", "science", "professionalism", "community care", "health custodians" and "doctoring" in order to conceal the greed, lust, lies, oppression, genocide, occultism, racketeering and evil. This argument proves that the pharmaceutical/medical/industrial complex is more occultic (hidden evil) than the pornography industry.

THIS CHAPTER WILL PRESENT evidence of the utterly rotten and evil fruit borne by the pharmaceutical/medical/industrial complex.

SUFFER THE LITTLE CHILDREN
   To quote Jesus Christ:

"It were better for him that a millstone were hanged about his neck, and he cast into the sea, than that he should offend one of these little ones." (Luke 17:2 (KJV)).

When analyzing the crippling effect of abusive medicine on humans, one finds that perhaps the most severely damaged humans are fetuses, infants and children.

PRE—CONCEPTION

Baby girls are born with all the egg cells they will ever have, in other words they do not grow new egg cells during their life time. These eggs are fragile and are the seed of new human life. Chemicals and radiation are two of the most violent agents these egg cells can be exposed to. Slight damage to an egg may be amplified to a severe malfunction in the human, similar to the invisible damage to seeds which result in malfunctional plants. Once the eggs have been damaged it leads to major defects such as infertility, brain dysfunction, birth deformities and cancer, as well as "lesser" problems such as impaired immunity, impaired eyesight, skin disorders and a host of other common disorders of the human body and mind. But then, that is the purpose of the medical industry - sick people will swell the coffers of the gluttonous pharmaceutical trade even further.

Most pharmaceutical medicines (prescription and over-the counter) have the potential to damage the fragile egg cells. Radiation from X-rays are even more destructive at the level of the cell. Both these dangerous practices are sold to patients by the billions of times per year world wide. The devastation caused to the human egg pool is unimaginable.

The value and geographical distribution of pharmaceutical sales give some idea of how many humans are exposed to chemical drugs:

SIZE OF THE WORLD MARKET

The value of the world pharmaceutical market was estimated by the European Pharmaceutical Industry (EFPIA) at US$164.5 billion in 1989. The 1990 market was estimated at being between $ 174 billion and $ 186 billion. The major market areas were: North America, 33.0%; Western Europe, 31.9%; Asia, 25.4%; Latin America, 3.9%; Eastern Europe, 3.1%; Africa, 1.8%; and Australia 1.0%. Forecasts for the year 2000 suggest the global market could reach $330 billion.

THAT EQUALS MORE than US$50 per human per year! The billions of x-ray $'s are not even included in this figure.

EGG CELLS ARE NOT the only pre-conception victims of chemicals. Male sperm is damaged by a wide array of chemicals, including hormonal medicines and X-rays.

DAMAGED EGG CELLS and sperm are certainly involved when the bewildering increase in auto-immune diseases (where the immune system becomes aggressive and damages the host body) are observed, of which AIDS is the most sensational. These diseases are not only on the increase, but younger and younger humans are suffering from these diseases, and are incurring untold miseries from conditions like Lupus (tissue degeneration), Arthritis, Allergies, Multiple sclerosis (paralysis) and Colitis (colon disease resulting in removal of colon).

THERE IS no substance such as a "safe man-made" chemical. Only a person with perfect knowledge of God's creation would be able to assess all the implications of a chemical insult to a human. The known dimensions of humans are mechanical (as in bones and blood), chemical (as in vitamins), electronic (as in nerve impulses), magnetic (as in bone growth), hormonal (as in insulin), enzymatic (as in DNA repair), mental (as in thoughts), spiritual (as in conversing with God) and many others. The unknown dimensions are real, but beyond the current knowledge of humans in general. Any man-made substance could impact all or some of the known, as well as the unknown dimensions in the human. The total listed toxic effects (side effects) of medicines number over 1 400 000! Most medicines also contain chemical excipients such as colourants, sweeteners, binders, stabilizers, flavourants, fillers and many more. The interaction of these toxic effects with other chemicals and foods in the human environment is beyond calculation. Medicines are deliberately not even required to be tested for interactions with other chemicals before marketing.

MANY MEDICINES also result in an altered state of consciousness, meaning that the user will experience a reduced will power and decision making ability.

VERY FEW WOMEN and men (of child generating age) have not been exposed to multiple drugs which has altered their egg cells and sperm cells. All new offspring in the medicine era actually have "3" parents, namely mom, dad and the silent participant - the pharmaceutical/medical/industrial complex. Fortunately (for the unborn), 20% of industrial couples have fertility problems (due to chemical damage) and cannot generate a damaged baby (perhaps a mixed blessing).

IN THE WOMB
Having survived the pre-conception chemical obstacle course, the fetus now enters the most hazardous place on earth, the womb. The fetus is already awash with residues of disturbing hormones which the mother took as contraceptives and cortisone during her life.

DURING THE FIRST 2-6 weeks (the most vulnerable), before the mother is 100% sure that she is pregnant, she is probably taking one or more medicines which the pharmaceutical/medical/industrial complex has persuaded her to take.

THE FOLLOWING SUBSTANCES would most likely be found in her medicines cabinet: pain killers, antibiotics, mood enhancers, sleep inducers, laxatives, diuretics, anti- spasmodics, cortisone for skin conditions, and in many cases, asthma drugs.

ONCE THE FETUS is acknowledged (the mother discovers she is pregnant), the danger really sets in. The fetus faces three possibilities namely, miscarriage, abortion or pregnancy - leading to life.

ABORTION BY THE PHARMACEUTICAL/MEDICAL/INDUSTRIAL complex has a high probability of being invoked. Abortion accounts for more human deaths this century than all other forms of violence combined, including all the great wars this century.

IN FIRST WORLD countries a person wishing to abort a fetus will be state assisted by the pharmaceutical/medical/industrial complex, whilst a person wishing to assist a fellow human suffering from cancer, by providing Vitamin B17 (Laetrile), will be arrested for "health fraud" (Vitamin B17 is a well proven agent in the arresting of some forms of cancer. The hand of Satan is unmistakable because:

"FOR WHOSO FINDETH **me findeth life, and shall obtain favour of the LORD. But he that sinneth against me wrongeth his own soul: <u>all they that hate me love death.</u>**" (Proverbs 8:35-36 (KJV)).

FROM THE ABOVE, God says "All those who hate God love death". Guess who performs most of the abortions? The medical industry of course! They are <u>trained</u> at university to do it! An estimated 20 000 000 babies are murdered by doctors every year! Has the medical industry staged a mass protest? No, because it is part of Satan's team effort in "seeking whom he may devour".

SHOULD the mother choose not to have an abortion she will enter the most horrendous form of "intensive care" invented by the medical industry. The medical industry has taken a God created process, namely birth, and has turned it into a lucrative mega-dollar industry. Women of all races, for thousands of years, have attended to the mostly traumatic and wonderful process of pregnancy and birthing, as ordained by God. No man, or woman can possibly understand all the complexities of the pregnancy and birth process. At least women <u>experience</u> childbirth. But what do women know (sic)? Doctor's know best!

HOME BIRTHING CAN NOW BE a criminal offense in some first world countries like Australia. The medical industry has legislated for the babies to be born inside the temples of Moloch (hospitals), where the proper sacrificial rites can be enforced and appropriate damage inflicted to ensure lucrative future customers for the medical industry. The reader will by now realize that a human is only useful to the medical industry if one is alive and sick. Neither dead nor well people are of any use to the medical industry, except for lucrative organ transplants, blood transfusions, skin grafts, bone marrow transplants and the like. This also accounts for the draconian, heroic efforts performed in life-saving technology of the medical industry. They are not driven by love, but by greed to save the goose that lays the golden eggs. The ideal status of a human for the pharmaceutical/medical/industrial complex, is for the human to remain in a limbo of being sick and alive.

DURING THE PREGNANCY, the mother and fetus will be coerced to subject themselves to the following harrowing health insults:

TESTS for the mother - Blood pressure, high or low:
 -Blood sugar, high or low
 -Urine proteins high
 -Blood iron, high or low
 -Urine immune activity

THIS BATTERY of tests is designed to find something dangerously "abnormal" which will eventually lead to a prescription for automatic repeat "check ups", probably a drug or more and maybe surgery.

Tests for the fetus - Ultrasound Scans (useless, unreliable and dangerous).
- Ultrasound foetal Monitoring During Labour (useless, unreliable and dangerous).
- AFP Tests (Alpha-fetoprotein) for Down's Syndrome. (Highly suspect, unreliable, false results leads to abortions).
- Chorionic Villus Sampling (for Down's Syndrome. Unreliable and dangerous).
- Amniocentesis (for Down's Syndrome. Causes club foot and miscarriage).

These tests result in physical, electronic, x-ray (semi-magnetic) and vibrational damage to the fetus. The tests are also unreliable, resulting in both false-positive as well as false-negative results. The technology is complex and requires high levels of operational skill as well as maintenance skills, both of which regularly fail. But, the tests are lucrative and each test results in a financial transaction somewhere! The insisting doctor will often be found to have shares in the equipment or receive a "kick-back" incentive from the owners of the equipment.

These tests are simply forms of divination and prognostication, to "see" into the future gender and biochemical status of the child. The Scriptural implications of using these occultic methods were stated in chapter 1.

What could the motive be for a person to be persuaded to test for a Down's Syndrome baby? It could only be for prognostication or for abortion! Nothing else.

What would God say about killing a Down's Syndrome baby?

"Yea, they sacrificed their sons and their daughters unto devils, And shed innocent blood, *even* the blood of their sons and of their daughters, whom they sacrificed unto the idols of Canaan: and the land was polluted with blood. Thus were they defiled with their own works, and went a whoring with their own inventions. Therefore was the wrath of the LORD kindled against his people, insomuch that he abhorred his own inheritance. And he gave them into the hand of the heathen; and they that hated them ruled over them." (Psalm 106:37-41. (KJV)).

The fetus, having survived this far (sort of), is then subjected to the doctor's pedestrian insults related to nutrition. God knows that bacteria (germs) flourish in iron rich environments. As designed in divine wisdom by God, pregnant women become anemic in order to reduce infection risk. Also, the expanded blood volume of the pregnant woman, which is a healthy sign, results in diluted iron concentrations and low blood pressure. Doctor's think otherwise, exactly the opposite to what God designed! Pregnant women are automatically placed on high iron supplements by doctor's to "counteract" anemia. The result is a pregnant woman with typical toxicity caused by synthetic iron, namely constipation and vaginal infections, at the very least. More serious toxicity caused by iron is common, such as premature births and small-for-date babies. Medical industry vitamin supplements are abominable concoctions of wrong ratios and toxic additives. This of course presents a brand new opportunity to treat the victim with a plethora of medicines to counteract the constipation and infections, which poisons the fetus and mother even further, which presents a brand new opportunity to treat the victim with a plethora of medicines, etc! The mother and infant have entered the vicious spiraling vortex of medical "supervision" and "care".

"Be sober, be vigilant, because your adversary the devil, as a roaring lion, walketh about, seeking whom he may devour". (1 Peter 5:8 (KJV))

The "devouring" is at it's most disgusting when infants and the unborn are the targets.

"Body stripping" for organs, as well as the use of, and the sale of placentas to the cosmetics industry is big international business for the medical industry. Brain damaged children are kept alive artificially, awaiting the negotiations around the sale of the child's organs. In the chain of command, the doctor can be likened as: "The highly trained medical professional is like an accessory to the vast pharmaceutical and health-care industries, as a stewardess is to a jet airliner and the aviation industry."
Ross Scholes: New Zealand health writer.

In his book "How to Raise a Healthy Child in Spite of your Doctor", Dr. Robert S Mendelsohn, an honest to God pediatrician (doctor of infants), has exposed hundreds of lies, fallacies, myths, errors, horrors and facts about his profession. He finally concludes that the greatest danger for the health of a child is the medical industry!

Dr. Francisco Contreras, surgical oncologist (specialist cancer surgeon) echoes these sentiments by stating that the greatest threats to human health are the medical industry, food industry, chemical industry and the regulatory authorities (government). Of course, in the roll-up pyramid of who governs the world, these four industries are different departments of the same owners.

THE BIRTH CONFINEMENT

The anti-God philosophy of the medical industry is absolutely evident in the birthing process. God created the human birthing process – the medical industry have perverted it beyond the wildest realms of greed, dependence-induction and de-powerment.

To realize the full horror of the "fruit" produced by the medical birthing industry, it helps to read a detailed description of the process by a specialist from inside the "obs/gyn", obstetrics and gynecology (birthing and infant doctors) speciality. Following is such a description:

(EMPHASIS AND BRACKETED comments by author).

WOMEN WOULD FIND HAVING babies a lot less painful, risky, and demeaning if the **obstetrical specialty were simply abolished**. Except for a handful of doctors who encourage natural birth, obstetricians are guilty of perpetuating an **unhealthy unscientific medical disgrace**. As you know by now, I have a low regard for Modern Medicine in general, but obstetrics sets my teeth on edge. It is the only medical specialty in which **almost everything** that the doctor does is medically indefensible and terribly wrong.

I SAID EARLIER that doctors have converted pregnancy, a natural, normal, inspiring physiological event – into a nine month disease. This sounds like a radical concept until you explore the machinations that preceded the creation of the medical specialty.

THROUGHOUT MOST OF human history babies were delivered by their mothers, not by doctors, with a female relative or a midwife standing by. **Midwives still assist most mothers in many of the most advanced nations in the world. Their success, in terms of infant and maternal mortality, surpasses that of American obstetricians,** who have distorted childbirth with **ritual procedures** that endanger both mother and child. Obstetricians also deny mothers and fathers the joy that natural childbirth should provide.

AMERICAN OBSTETRICAL PRACTICE is flawed because its **roots are not in medical science,** but in historical nonsense, male-ego, and plain old-fashioned **greed**. It originated in Europe, when the eighteenth-century male barber-surgeons realized that they were losing countless opportunities to increase their income and began plotting to take childbirth away from midwives. It wasn't easy to do, because midwives were quite capable of assisting at childbirth and had been demonstrating this capability for thousands of years. True, maternal and infant mortalities were then tragically frequent, as today's obstetricians are fond of pointing out, but only because Ignaz Semmelweis had not yet demonstrated that infections are caused by germs passed from doctors to mothers. Conveniently forgotten is the fact that maternal and infant death rates doubled when the barber surgeons got into the act. Hospitalized mothers got childbed fever because the doctors rushed from sick beds and autopsies to deliveries without bothering to wash their hands. The doctors had no excuse to co-opt childbirth as long as it was perceived as a non medical physiological function that mothers could accomplish themselves with little more than emotional support. In order to get their hands on all those patients, the **doctors had to convert childbirth into a disease**.

THEY DID it by interfering with the natural process and creating medical interventions that only they could perform. As insurance, they **defamed the midwives, branding them as witches when they lost mothers or babies and having them tortured or burned at the stake (the church rendered able assistance; author)**. The first witch hanged in the American colonies was a midwife whom the doctors accused. A landmark event in the doctors' long campaign to take over childbirth was the invention of the Forceps by Peter Chamberlen in 1588. He and three generations of his family won acclaim for handling difficult deliveries by using a primitive version of this now abused and overused tool. They kept the **device a secret** from other doctors - and from mothers, too - by working under a sheet and carrying their forceps around in a locked wooden box. This instrument was the obstetricians first leap into technology, hailed by them as proof of their superiority over the midwives. **No one kept score how often it mangled soft tiny heads**. Chamberlen set a pattern for technological intervention - and for its adverse consequences - that dominates obstetrical practice in the United States today. Obstetricians should build him a shrine and pay him homage every time they go to the bank.

THE FORCEPS, however, was not the obstetrical breakthrough that finally took the process of childbirth away from the midwives -and from mothers, as well. The turning point was the **elimination of the birthing stool**, on which mothers delivered babies by allowing natural contractions and gravity to do their work. Doctors began placing mothers flat on their backs on high tables with their knees raised. This made it virtually impossible to deliver their own babies and assured that they would need a doctor to help.

"AND HE SAID, When ye do the office of a midwife to the Hebrew women, and see *them* upon the stools; if it *be* a son, then ye shall kill him: but if it *be* a daughter, then she shall live. But the midwives feared God, and did not as the king of Egypt commanded them, but saved the men children alive." (Exodus 1:16-17 (KJV)).

SCRIPTURE SEEMS to indicate that even the ancients knew how God planned for the machinations of gravity and attendance of official midwives, to take care of birthing.

THE SUPINE LITHOTOMY (laying down) position is the basis for most of the intervention that is routine in modern obstetrical practice. It has effectively **deprived women** of all **control** over their childbirth. It has also made having babies infinitely more difficult, perilous, and painful, and provided obstetricians with seemingly countless rational reasons to come to the mother's aid. As a doctor once commented in The Journal of Pediatrics, obstetricians are like firemen. They both rescue people - the only difference is that the firemen don't start their own fires!

CONSIDERING the radical nature of the change from the birthing stool to the supine position, you would assume that it evolved from cautious scientific research. Incredibly, it didn't.

THE PRACTICE of laying birthing mothers flat on their backs was initiated to **satisfy a kinky erotic aberration of France's Louis XIV.**

KING LOUIS IT SEEMS, got his kicks by peering from behind a curtain while his mistresses, of whom there were many, gave birth. He was frustrated because his vision was obscured when the women were seated on birthing stools. In an inspired moment he used his royal clout to persuade a male midwife to improve his view. A woman was placed on a high, flat table, with her knees up, and King Louis was immensely pleased with the result.

NOT SURPRISINGLY, other doctors soon concluded that what was good enough for the royal household must also be good for everyone else. They adopted the lithotomy position, apparently in the belief that Newton and Kepler were wrong, and that by royal edict the law of gravity had been repealed.

THAT EPISODE MIGHT BE AMUSING as a footnote to medical history were it not for this ridiculous position by obstetricians delivering babies today. The only refinement that has been added is one that Louis himself might have appreciated but that mothers certainly don't - the use of stirrups that keep the mother's legs strapped in place. The lithotomy position cannot be defended for any reason other than the doctor's convenience. From the mother's agonizing perspective the delivery could be made more difficult only if she were hung up by her heels.

WAY back in 1933 Mengert and Murphy, in an extensive experimental study, recorded intra-abdominal pressure at the height of maximum straining effort during labor. Their research involved more than 1,000 observations of women placed in seven postures. They found that the greatest pressure was exerted in the sitting position. This was due to measured visceral weight and increased muscular efficiency. In 1937, another researcher presented x-rays and measurements that indicated that squatting alters the pelvic shape that makes it advantageous for delivery. I know of no study that has ever negated this evidence that women should not be confined to the supine position during labor. Yet with few exceptions, women in labor in the United States are still placed flat on their backs with their feet in stirrups.

SINCE IT OBVIOUSLY HAS NO legitimate medical basis, you are entitled to ask why doctors continue to force mothers to have their babies while strapped down flat on their backs. In the absence of all any other rational explanation, I will give you the only answer that makes any sense. The position itself creates the pathology that makes normal births abnormal and provides about 95% of his reason to exist.

THE TRAUMA that the doctor has **created** provides him with a succession of **opportunities to appear necessary** and to satisfy his desire to intervene. Meanwhile, the mother has become a bit player in the drama of her own child's birth, and the father is lucky if he is even allowed to be one of the props in the scene.

THE PREGNANT WOMAN'S troubles often begin even before she enters the hospital. Although she and her husband may have violated the speed limit to get there because her contractions were frequent and strong, they often slow down abruptly - or even stop - the moment she walks up to the hospital door. This reaction is so common that it even has a name - uterine inertia - and those who have studied it believe it is the result of **fear**.

WHEN SHE ENTERS THE HOSPITAL, the mother's apprehension escalates because she immediately loses the support of her husband. She is placed in a wheelchair and trundled off to the labor room, leaving her husband behind at the admission desk. He can't go because he is needed for the hospital's most important rite – assuring the business office that he will be able to pay the bill.

ANY DOCTOR who is not blinded by his own training and prejudice knows that labor is prolonged and made more difficult and painful by fear. I have had the pleasure of observing - even in my own daughters - the relaxed, rewarding experience that an undrugged natural home birth can be. Fear is neutralized by comfortable, familiar surroundings and the support of family and friends. Yet virtually every aspect of modern obstetrical practice conspires to isolate the mother in unfamiliar surroundings and increase her apprehension.

THE LABOR ROOM to which the mother is sent has all the appeal of a prison cell, and for all practical purposes that is what it becomes. The typical bare, dismal cubicle is scarcely large enough to contain a metal washstand and a hospital bed. Separated from her husband, the mother stands there frightened and alone, obeying commands from an overworked and often indifferent and impatient nurse. She is told to strip and slip into an ill fitting hospital gown that ties with strings and flops open in the back, doing nothing to improve her morale. Then she is ordered to climb into bed.

THAT SEEMINGLY INNOCUOUS act seals her fate, for until she is moved to the delivery room she will be confined to her bed. She will be denied the freedom of movement and exercise that would relieve her tensions, ease her fears, expedite her labor, and reduce or eliminate her pain. Her baby will be exposed to the **risk of damage or death** from **lack of nutrition and oxygen** that the supine position may cause, and the hazards that will result from its mother's treatment with drugs. The mother's pain will be increased, so **drugs will be administered** that will retard and prolong labor. Labor will be induced by invading the uterus and **rupturing the membranes**, increasing the risk of infection and fetal damage or death. The mother will be further confined by attachment of intravenous gadgetry to keep a vein open for **administration of drugs** and to provide nourishment because she will not be allowed to eat or drink. A fetal monitor will be strapped to her abdomen or inserted into her uterus and **screwed into the baby's scalp**, to monitor the fetal trauma that the obstetrician's intervention may well induce. Ultimately, and usually for the convenience of the doctor, oxytocin will be administered to expedite labor, resulting in tetanic (and titanic) contractions so strong that they may **injure the fetus**. The mother's pain, which escalates because of the way she is being treated, becomes so unbearable that pain killing injections are given that paralyze the lower half of her body. The mother can no longer feel her contractions and must be told when to push.

FINALLY THE POOR woman is moved to the delivery room, strapped into stirrups, and an episiotomy is performed. The **doctor** delivers the baby because the **mother is no longer able to do** it, and more often than not he will use forceps because he is unwilling to wait for nature to take its course.

This concludes the mother's experience with the "miracle of birth"

THE DOCTOR hurriedly cuts the cord before it has stopped pulsating, so that the infant's blood backs up in the mother. It is that mixing that produces erythroblastosis (Rh disease) in a **subsequent child**. He tugs on the cord to expedite delivery of the placenta, **increasing the mother's risk** of hemorrhage and possibly leaving some pieces behind. He must then **invade the uterus** to capture the fragments. The mother's **risk of infection**, already increased over the previous hours by multiple vaginal examinations, becomes even greater. Next he must repair the damage done to the perineum (outer part of vagina) by the episiotomy (surgery to enlarge the vagina orifice) he performed. As I will explain later, this may cause **sexual dysfunction** later on. Finally, in denial of everything that prompted the mother to go through this ordeal, the baby is whisked off to the newborn nursery, and mother to the recovery room to sleep off the drugs.

THIS IS MOTHERHOOD?
  This is medicine?"

THE HORRIBLE DAMAGE has only just started. For brevity, some of the other diabolical insults invented by the medical industry, and foisted on the mother and child during birthing, are summarized:

MEDICAL ACTION: **NEGATIVE RESULT**
  MA: Shaving of pubic hair.
  NR: Triple risk of infection.
  MA: Fetal heart monitor.
  NR: Death, brain damage, etc.
  MA: 19 Different drugs used during pregnancy and delivery.
  NR: Hundreds of toxic and permanent unwanted effects.
  MA: Birthing tranquilisers, sedatives, caudals (rectals), epidurals, saddle blocks, paracervical blocks, spinals and anestehtics.
  NR: Physical and intellectual damage to both mother and child.

MA: Induction of labour.

NR: Brain damage.

MA: Episiotomomy (vagina cut).

NR: Infection, slow healing, permanent sexual dysfunction, accidents to baby's brain.

MA: Ceasarean. (A vast lie and scam). Most "emergency" ceasareans are performed during office hours, proving that there was no emergency.

NR: Completely un-Godly. The birth canal performs vital life long functions. The baby is robbed of this natural process.

MA: Silver nitrate eye drops or antibiotic drops in eyes.

NR: Astigmatism and myopia, blocked tear ducts, conjunctivitis. (Permanent and some temporary eye disorders).

MA: Vitamin K injections.

NR: Cancer (especially leukemia), jaundice, which leads to dangerous ultraviolet bilirubin light treatment, which leads to more treatment.

MA: Anti-psychotic drugs to promote breast milk. (one of the toxic strange side effects is abnormal production of breast milk) (sulpiride, Sulparex, Eglonyl).

NR: This must rate as one of the best examples of perverse medical dementia. The drug is semi-lethal and is employed for it's toxic side-effect to produce milk.

THE BABY HAS NOT YET LEFT hospital and is already damaged for life.

THE FIRST 18 MONTHS

If the baby is still alive, it will be subjected to some of the worst chemical and health insults imaginable. These insults include synthetic, denatured formula milk, vaccinations and antibiotics. All three of these medical abominations cause life-long damage and are based on the false science described in chapter 5.

FORMULA MILK CONTAINS TOO much iron and is guaranteed to cause bacterial infections. Mothers milk contains very little iron and then in a different form. The devilish lie of the formula milk manufacturers is easy to expose – they claim to copy mothers milk – then why do they insist on adding something that is not in mothers milk? In their scientific wisdom they omit certain essential nutrients found in breast milk such as DHA (docosahexaoenioic acid) and other oils required for proper brain development. Maybe improving God's work? Doctors had promoted formula milk for decades before they had to bow their "science" to the common sense of the people. The error was so obvious and glaring that it is at least one lie that was unsustainable.

SOME OF THE implications of formula milk are:

LOW IMMUNITY due to absence of breast milk antibodies.
   Allergies due to intolerance to dairy, soya and grains.
   Mucous forming leads to ear and digestive canal infections.
   Permanent infections and constipation from iron overload.

ONCE THE BABY has developed serious infections from the use of formula milk, the doctor will automatically prescribe antibiotics. Most formula manufacturers are owned by the subsidiaries and nominees of the pharmaceutical/medical/industrial complex! The reader can contemplate the implications of the instance where the same agent is causing the problem (milk formula branch) and offering the solution (anti-biotic branch). To the ruthless servants of Mammon, this is considered "creative marketing".

ANTIBIOTIC USE by infants hold the following horrendous risks:
   Massive increase in DNA mutation (meaning damage to inherited genes)
   Diabetes
   Hearing defects
   Digestive ecology destruction (leading to maldigestion and malnutrition)
   Resistant strains of germs (creating devilish super bugs in the infant patient)

ALL TYPES of diseases can then flow from these complications because most of the complications cause damage to the immune system. The medical industry has created a veritable "self perpetuating" gold fountain. The only possible threat to this vicious and greed driven arrangement, develops if the customers die or, against all odds, become healthy.

BETWEEN THE FIRST day of birth and 72 months of age, the child is subjected to one of the most devastating immune insults imaginable, namely a barrage of vaccinations. The pharmaceutical/medical/industrial complex must rank immunization as one of the flagship deceptions they have foisted on humans. The deception could not have been developed without the evolution theory and Pasteur's "germ" theory of disease. It is on this false foundation that vaccination and immunization have been sold to gullible victims worldwide, including, and especially, third world countries.

FOR A SUMMARY OF THE ABOMINATION, the back cover of a succinct book sums it up:

DID YOU KNOW?

THE U.S. GOVERNMENT keeps a **secret** list of several thousand people who were **damaged or killed** by vaccines?

AUTHORITIES REFUSE to investigate correlations between vaccines and several new diseases?

MEDICAL POLICYMAKERS ARE PLANNING to squirt their "magic bullet" supervaccine into your **child's mouth**?

TAKE a trip into the shadowy underworld of **vaccine theory**, where **live** viruses are brewed in diseased animal organs prior to being "stabilized" with **chemical compounds** and **carcinogenic (cancer causing) substances**, prior to being **injected into your healthy child.** Then take a look behind the scenes at vaccine reality, where **thousands of children are damaged and killed every year**, where Persian Gulf War patriots are freely experimented on, and where **human genetic patterns are altered indiscriminately.** These stories and more are revealed in this profound **expose on vaccinations.**

Every physician knows (Author: **no, they don't.**) vaccines can **maim and kill patients.** Neil Miller brings the dangers and horrors of forced immunizations out of the closet . What he reveals will scare the hell out of you. - Alan Cantwell, M.D., author, AIDS and the Doctors of Death.

The USA is world renowned for its **appalling infant mortality rate.** If anything should be compulsory in the United States, it is the reading of this book by every politician, medical doctor, parent and citizen. - Viera Scheibner, Ph.D., principal research scientist.

In order to understand how people could be duped into believing such treachery, the underlying rationale of vaccination and antibiotics needs to be scrutinized in terms of various lies. The first lie is the germ theory lie.

THE GERM THEORY LIE:

Perhaps the most successful lie of the medical industry is the "germ theory" of Pasteur. It is second only to the lie by Darwin's followers. For the medical industry to instill fear of disease into patients, this abominable theory is essential. Once healthy patients realize that there is almost nothing to fear from germs, and that the "germ killing magic bullet" of the doctor is an illusion, the whole medical industry marketing paradigm falls apart. It is the germ theory, and the apparent early success of antibiotics, which have escalated the image of the medical industry from caring professionals, into glitzy high-tech wizards, as portrayed by their marketing hype.

FOR THE GERM theory to stand, a foundation of other lies has to be in place, or else the germ theory house of cards will collapse. These other lies which are required are: the evolution theory or Darwinism, the "magic bullet" theory, and the "bad god" theory.

1. NEO-DARWINISM IS REQUIRED BECAUSE:

"THE GERM THEORY of disease developed during the gory phase of Darwinism, when the interplay between living things was regarded as a struggle for survival . . . This attitude moulded from the beginning the pattern of all the attempts at the control of microbial disease. It led to a kind of aggressive war against the microbes, aimed at their elimination from the sick individual and from the community. No place here for the biological concepts now prevailing in other fields of natural history . . . The view that some sort of biological equilibrium can be achieved between the microbes and their potential victims has not been popular among physicians and medical scientists".

PROFESSOR RENÉ DUBOS. *Mirage of Health; 1960*
This false idea is necessary because the "survival struggle" of the "evolution theory" requires germs to threaten humans, so that "natural selection" can take place, to "evolve" the human species.

2. THE "MAGIC BULLET" theory is required because:

A MEDICAL INDUSTRY doctor is required to administer the antibiotic which was known as a magic bullet in the early days of antibiotics. The patient cannot perform self-treatment, or go to a natural healer or heal and protect themselves by other means. So the medical industry invented a terrible threat "out there" called "germs" who only they could detect and kill, and thus become "angels of light in white coats" which saved and protected humans against the invisible germs. Only a "licensed" doctor may administer the germ killing medicines, by law.

3. The "bad god" theory is required because: (paraphrasing Dr. Mendelsohn). It states that the god who created these "bad", disease causing germs, cannot possibly be a good god. So by joining the "new scientific" religion one can join forces with a "good" god whose medicines will kill the pesky germs of the old "bad" god. Voila, the God of creation is replaced with the god of science.

To make the complex deception more acceptable to medical students, a set of impressive scientific doctrines, called Koch's postulates, had to be invented and propagated.

THE DOCTRINE STATES THAT: For a specific bacteria (or germ) to be the cause of a disease, it must:
1) be found in every case of the disease,
2) not be found when the disease is not present,
3) be able to exist outside the tissues of the host; and
4) produce the disease when the host is exposed to it.

THE FIRST OF Koch's postulates is **false** since scientists now know that specific microorganisms are not found in each case of the disease. The second of Koch's postulates is **false** because germs are consistently found in the bodies of animals and people who show no signs of any disease The third postulate is **false** because many germs depend on animal or human organisms for their survival and cannot survive outside the tissues. Finally, the fourth postulate is **false** because studies indicate that many people will not contract a particular disease, even when thoroughly exposed to its "disease germ".

THE OBVIOUS DECEPTION of the germ theory can be seen from the simple question: If germs caused disease, why is everyone who is exposed to the germs, not sick?

One of the most bizarre practices in the "medical germ circus" is the use of stethoscopes (heart beat meters) and blood pressure meters. One can observe all the every day draconian germ killing procedures employed in the medical settings such as the surgery, hospital, nursery and laboratories. Then one can puzzle about why the doctor's never clean their official badges (stethoscope), which is visible around the collar or peeping from the white coat pocket. The doctor's dog has probably been slavering on the stethoscope in the back of the doctor's Mercedes. The stethoscope is carried from one sick patient to the next, to the cafeteria, toilet, the car and home. If there are dangerous germs, this is where they will be, in a grand assortment. The same goes for the blood pressure meters toted from one patient to the next. If germs were mobile, these would be their ideal vehicles. The reason why this anomaly exists is because of the "infallibility" of the "angel of light" – namely that all these horrible germs can only exist on other people, not on doctor's, or their car, children, dog, stethoscope, etc. Medical staff, who have the greatest exposure to germs, do not suffer exceptionally high infection rates, proving once more that germs do not cause disease.

Yet this patently false dogma is taught to medical industry students around the world. When a person dedicates their life to the work of Satan (for instance the hippocratic oath), then Scripture states that, in the latter days:

"But evil men and seducers shall wax worse and worse, deceiving, and being deceived." (2 Timothy 3:13. (KJV)).

Included in the manufacture of vaccines are: Carcinogens (cancer agents) and toxic substances such as germs, aluminum (a neuro-toxin), live viruses, Thimerosal (a Mercury derivative), bacteria, formaldehyde (a major component of embalming fluid), animal RNA and DNA, monkey kidneys, foreign proteins, calf serum, chick embryo, undetected animal viruses, all being squirted into a HEALTHY BABY.

The result is that millions of people are crippled, killed, damaged, impaired, maimed and deceived by the medical industry when immunization is foisted on them. And it is sold to people worldwide although it is based on a completely false foundation.

THERE IS A MORE sinister aspect to vaccination as well:

WHAT HAPPENS NEXT, once this foul concoction - live viruses, bacteria, toxic substances, and diseased animal matter - is created?

THIS WITCH'S brew is forced into the healthy child.

SATANIC RITUALS:
Dr. Robert Mendelsohn often criticized modern medicine for its sanctimonious doctrine. He argued that "**doctors are the priests who dispense holy water** in the form of inoculations" to ritually initiate our loyalty into the larger medical industry. Dr Richard Moskowitz agrees: "Vaccines have become **sacraments of our faith** in biotechnology. Their efficacy and safety are widely seen as self-evident and needing no further proof."

OTHERS SEE a link between vaccinations and **Satanic rituals** or **witchcraft**, where animals are sacrificed and their organs brewed in a hellish concoction of horrid substances : **voodoo medicine** by 20th century mad scientists. Sadly, our children are their unwilling subjects as society is slowly devoured by their insatiable appetite for human experimentation.

CHILDREN CAN BE VACCINATED with up to 36 different vaccinations during their first 60 months.

SCIENCE INDEED! It is the science of Satan, no less.

1 ½ YEARS TO PUBERTY:

The biggest health threat which children face in this period, is from wrong diet, antibiotics and behavior altering drugs. They will also have their tonsils (integral component of the immune system) butchered out as a routine procedure.

THE FOOD INDUSTRY will see to it that the child is seduced into eating a diet consisting of mostly processed foods, consisting mainly of refined starches. The dietetics profession, being "temple prostitutes" to both the medical industry and the food industry, will echo the marketing strategies of both industries to the child and the mother. (The dietitians are normally trained inside the medical faculties of universities, and the dietetics curriculum is dictated by the food industry).

NUTRITION IS SIMPLY the most vital aspect of human health (Chapter 11 elaborates on this subject. The curriculum of the doctor contains a zero application in nutrition, meaning that the doctor is not trained in real nutrition at all! It is patently obvious that the doctors are not trained to promote health knowledge, if they were, then nutrition would have been their major subject! The dietitians are trained to sell big business processed foods (disease causing) and the doctor is trained to treat disease symptoms (health avoidance). What a perfect trap for the multitudes! Could humans have developed such diabolical systems? Maybe, but only with dictates from Lucifer and some of his officers, Moloch, Mammon and Baal.

"**No man can serve two masters: for either he will hate the one, and love the other; or else he will hold to the one, and despise the other. <u>Ye cannot serve God and mammon.</u>**" (Matthew 6:24 (KJV)).

THIS STATEMENT by Jesus raises an interesting question? What does the statement then make of the servant (doctor) who serves the medical industry, which in turn serves Mammon, all in the same chain of command? The medical industry serves mammon, no doubt, but what about the servants of the medical industry? Similarly, people working in the pornography industry as an administrative employee for instance, should ask themselves whether they want to be party to the goals of the pornography industry. The question arises then whether the servant of the servant of Satan bears any responsibility?

THE AVERAGE WESTERN child will be insulted with about 36 courses of antibiotics before the child has reached puberty. The cavalier application of antibiotics by doctors also rests on the germ theory and the "magic bullet" theory mentioned earlier in the chapter.

ANTIBIOTICS CAN CAUSE every known disease because it disrupts the 400+ species of friendly, God created, germs on which human life is totally dependent (known as symbiotic micro-flora and microbes or probiotics). All dangerous germs can be simply contained by following the hygiene rules in the Bible, particularly Leviticus. Dr. Paul Brand (surgeon and leprosy researcher) who wrote "Fearfully and Wonderfully Made", stated that no one has ever improved on the germ management rules of the Bible. God created the human ecology and provided the "handbook" of how to keep it healthy. The pharmaceutical/medical/industrial complex created man-made antibiotics which have since ruined human immunity and have forced disease related germs to defend themselves by becoming "superbugs".

THERE ARE RARE, serious and/or life threatening conditions for which antibiotics can be useful. The pharmaceutical/medical/industrial complex has abused the use of antibiotics beyond imagination. It has reached the situation where more diseases are caused by antibiotics than anything else on earth, (malnutrition excepted).

BY THE TIME the typical youngsters start attending school, they are so damaged by the medical industry abuses that they have suffered brain malfunction. Trapped between a junk food diet and biochemical chaos caused by medicines, the biochemical status of the child is unfit for paying attention, learning or concentrating. These "syndromes" are then given medical industry names such as Attention Deficit Syndrome or Hyperactivity Syndrome. Opportunity for more money now lurks for both the medical industry and their "psychobabbling" colleagues in the Psychology/ Psychiatry industry.

THE CHILD WILL THEN BE SUBJECTED to a brand new chemical insult, namely psychostimulants. These drugs result in alleged improvement in concentration and/or hyperactivity. Some of the implications researched by a caring psychiatrist are listed below:

THE IDEA that Ritalin or **other stimulants** correct biochemical imbalances in the brain of hyperactive children, although promoted by Wender and others, is **false on two counts** : First there is no known chemical imbalance in these children, and second, it generally is accepted that Ritalin has the same effect on all individuals, regardless of their psychiatric diagnosis or behavior.

FREQUENTLY LISTED as **side effects** are sadness or **depression**, social withdrawal, **flattened emotions**, and loss of energy.

CONSISTENT with the **brain-disabling** principle of biopsychiatric treatment (chapter 3). I believe that these subduing effects are **not side effects but the primary therapeutic effect, rendering the child less troublesome and easier to manage.**

OTHER NEGATIVE EFFECTS of Ritalin include **growth suppression**, tics, skin rashes, nausea, headache, stomach ache, and **psychosis**.

ABNORMAL MOVEMENTS, such as tics and spasms, sometimes develop. Many cases of full blown Tourette's Syndrome are reported, characterized by both facial and vocal tics.

Sometimes these neurological disorders do not subside after termination of treatment, and tragically, neuroleptics may be prescribed to control them, increasing the risk of further neurological disorders.

FREQUENTLY THE CLINICAL effect is mixed, quieting the child during the day but causing insomnia at night, or producing up-and-down cycles. Also, Ritalin can make a child more irritable rather than calmer.

MILLIONS OF CHILDREN are forced onto these drugs by the medical industry, in cohort with desperate teachers and psychological counselors. These stimulants are addictive and the child will seek a replacement narcotic when the school medicines are stopped, maybe non-prescription drugs like cannabis (dope)?

BY NOW, the child is being dragged deeper and deeper into the demonised vortex of biochemical destruction.

AT THIS POINT the parent(s) may be introduced to the medical industry gambit known as "blame the victim". The psychobabblers will attempt to blame the parent's and/or the child's "attitude" or "psyche" for the ADD (Attention deficit disorder). Maybe the child and/or parents are coerced into psychotherapy sessions where they are prepared for a long, expensive and deceptive course, which results in guilt laden, confused people. Satan could not do it better himself!

THE TEENAGE YEARS:
Hormonal disturbances, acne, asthma, sinusitis, appendicitis, venereal disease, mood disorders and obesity offer the medical industry ample scope for not losing it's grip on the customer (victim).

ACNE PRESENTS OPPORTUNITIES for applying two of the most vicious medicines yet devised. Continuous antibiotics for months on end, and/or a form of synthetic Vitamin A that is lethal to the fetus. These children all develop major health problems decades after they have suffered this violent form of chemical abuse. Teenage girls are routinely placed on oral contraceptives to control acne – a real invitation to promiscuity.

THE YOUNG MARRIED LIFE:

Infertility, contraception, female dysfunction and, of course, a brand new crop of babies. The onset of digestive disorders such as "spastic colon", start surfacing at this stage after 2- 3 decades of processed foods. This, and young adulthood, is probably the least lucrative stage (for the medical industry), of the victim's life.

THE MIDDLE YEARS:

Things start looking up for the medical industry here. Cholesterol, hysterectomies, high blood pressure, chronic digestive disorders, kidney stones, gall bladder disease, and the early incidence of cancer all start increasing.

AFTER 60:

This is the gold at the end of the journey. Prostate disease, heart disease, cataracts, Alzheimer's, regular "check ups" and batteries of tests, serious digestive disorders and severe mood disorders are standard fare by this stage of life.

AFTER 80:

All that expensive, life saving technology can now be applied to people who would rather die. The enthusiasm of the medical industry to save the old folks is understandable. If the victim dies, the income source is gone! Most humans engage in top performance to protect their income, and doctor's must rank at the top of the income defenders. The fact that the expensive efforts are trotted out as Samaritan endeavors is only another deception. Performing lethal, expensive and useless surgery on octogenarians must rank as one of mammon's cruelest ploys. Not happy to interfere only with the very process of God's created life processes, the medical industry also interfere with the death process. The administrators of estates are astonished to find huge medical claims lodged against the deceased estate by the medical industry, all from the dying process. This is not assisting life, it is robbery of vulnerable old people and their gullible heirs.

"HONOR THY FATHER **and thy mother: that thy days may be long upon the land which the LORD thy God giveth thee."** (Exodus 20:12. (KJV)).

FOLLOWING ARE SOME MORE "FRUITS" from the pharmaceutical/medical/industrial tree:

THE TREATMENT: THE "FRUIT"
TT: Standard medical industry treatment in the USA.
TF: Iatrogenesis (doctor caused disease) kills 500 000 patients per year in the USA. The morbidity number (sickness caused) is unknown.
TT: Major cause of AIDS is medical treatment.
TF: All medicines disrupt immunity.
TT: General comments from Britain.
TF: Women are found to be given hysterectomies without their consent.
Pregnant women abort perfectly healthy babies after the fetus is wrongly diagnosed as being defective.
Some 1,000 cervical smear tests are misdiagnosed.
In one hospital district, nearly 2,000 patients are misdiagnosed as having cancer and given treatment that may increase their chances of developing the disease.
New evidence emerges about hormones containing Creutzfeld-Jacob disease (mad cows disease) in fertility treatments given to women.
Growth hormone was also found to be contaminated with CJD (see above).
Surgical patients are dying from bad care in hospital.
Complaints against doctors have tripled since 1977.

Half of all trainee doctors admit to major mistakes in giving intravenous drugs.

Drug prescriptions have gone up by 30 per cent in seven years.

13,000 British lives are lost a year because intensive-care patients aren't monitored properly.

AND THAT IS ONLY what is read in a morning paper in Britain in a single month in 1994.

TT: <u>Diagnoses</u>:
    Blood-pressure Readings
    Angiography
    X-rays
    Bone Scans
    CAT Scans
    MRI Scans
    Lab Tests
    'Oscopy' Tests
TF: **Partially or totally**:

Expensive, useless, inappropriate, dangerous, debilitating, inaccurate, prone to failure, not properly maintained, leukemia causing, unscientific.

TT: <u>Screening for cancer</u>:
    Smear tests
    Mammograms
    Screening ovarian cancer
    Prostate cancer screening
TF: **Partially or totally**:

Expensive, useless, inappropriate, dangerous, debilitating, inaccurate, prone to failure, not properly maintained, leukemia and cancer causing, unscientific, untrue, deadly, racketeering.

TT: <u>"Miracle Cures"</u>:
    Drug Testing on the Public.
    Data Torture (manipulating results).
    Too Much of a Good Thing.
    Asthma Drugs.

Steroids (including cortisone).
Drugs for Eczema.
Arthritis Drugs.
Drugs for Hypertension.
Combination Heart Drugs.
Drugs for Epilepsy.
Anti-depressants.
Chemotherapy.
Drugs to Treat the Side-effects of Drugs.
TF: According to the advertisements the doctor reads in the medical glossy literature.
Witnessed by withdrawal of 1000's of drugs from the market, many years after release.
Scientific fraud on large scale.
Antibiotics overprescribed 97% of the time.
Causes the disease.
The sleaziest of all harmful drugs.
As for steroids.
Damage far exceeds the small benefit.
Anything from useless to lethal. Makes blood pressure worse.
Increases heart attacks.
Lethal. Only useful in extremes.
Damage far exceeds the small benefit.
Causes cancer.
Damaging and lucrative.
TT: <u>Dental medicines:</u>
Amalgam fillings (mercury).
Fluoride supplements. *
TF: Ruins the immune system slowly.
Thyroid, bone and immune damage.

---

* FLUORIDE IS one of the most devastating substances ever forced on humans. Fluoride derivatives have far reaching mental and physical implications. The author ranks Fluoride in the "top ten" strategies by the pharmaceutical/medical/ industrial complex to destroy human health, and control behavior of the masses by insidious mind alteration. Fluoride is an active ingredient in some of the tricyclic antidepressants, of which Prozac is a best seller (related to tricyclics). A recent (September 1998) and exhaustive study, consisting of more than 300 pages, exposing the secret horrors of Fluoride, has been compiled by Stuart Thomson of Pharmapact, in South Africa. Food, water, pre-natal supplements, kiddies "teeth building" supplements, tooth paste, medicines and many other every day products are laced with this Satanic chemical. One of the characteristics of fluoride is to generate <u>docility</u> in the victim who ingests it. One of the chemical solutions for the state is to fluoridate drinking water in order to keep the masses docile.

WOMEN'S DISEASES, CANCER, AIDS AND HEART DISEASE:

These subjects deserve special mention because they constitute some of the most outrageous lies and practices in the pharmaceutical/medical/industrial complex.

WOMEN'S DISEASES:

The medical industry mistreats women so badly that a whole book has been compiled on the atrocities. One of the authors has inside information on the pharmaceutical/medical/industrial complex, since both her husband and father are doctors.

THE DUST COVER gives a glimpse of the book as follows:
Women's medical complaints are more than twice as likely as men's to be dismissed by doctors as psychosomatic.

90% of women with breast cancer are eligible for lumpectomies, yet more than half will undergo mastectomies.

NO DEFINITIVE RESEARCH exists about the long term safety of birth control pills, yet doctors have prescribed them to millions of women for decades.

TREATMENT FOR HEART DISEASE, the number one killer of women in this country, have been tested mainly on men.

Women with kidney failure are 30% less likely to receive kidney transplants than men.

IN THIRTY YEARS of research on treatments for alcoholism, only 8,000 of the 110,000 subjects studied were women.

ARMED WITH THESE STARK TRUTHS, "Outrageous Practices" investigates medical schools, where inflatable sex dolls are used to teach anatomy; explores research facilities where male doctors in their fifties are studying other male doctors in their fifties...

ONE RESEARCH SCIENTIST, a woman, has described Hormone Replacement Therapy and the contraceptive pill as "the biggest medical blunders of the century. (Not blunders, but strategies, more likely: author).

MILLIONS OF WOMEN are contracting gross diseases ranging from cancer to insanity as a result of hormonal chaos caused mainly by prescription drugs and surgery promoted by the medical industry. The diseases so caused are of course part of the "devouring" Satan is performing. The beneficiaries of the system are the pharmaceutical/medical/industrial complex and Satan.

CANCER:
One (or more) in three (industrialised) people are destined to get cancer. That means more than one out of three!

THE FOLLOWING INTRODUCTION to a book was written by a medical industry doctor who's wife and himself were subjected to standard medical industry cancer treatment:

DEDICATION...

TO MARCIA, MY FRIEND. AND MOTHER OF MY CHILDREN, WHO WAS **MUTILATED AND DESTROYED** BY THE FOUR HORSEMAN OF THE NEW APOCALYPSE...

* ORTHODOX MEDICINE *

* THE PHARMACEUTICAL INDUSTRY *

* THE FDA AND THE NIH * (**both are public service medicines and cancer authorities**).

* CITIZENS **AND INDUSTRIES** WHO DESECRATE OUR LIVES ON EARTH*
SHE DIED OF BRAIN CANCER **AFTER UNNECESSARY SURGERY AND HUMILIATING AND NOXIOUS RADIATION.**

DOES one see accountants turning against their own profession like this? The most severe critics of the system are from within! Brave pioneers indeed.

"YE SERPENTS, **ye generation of vipers, how can ye escape the damnation of hell?**" (Matthew 23:33. (KJV)).

CHRIST CALLED them by their proper name. He did not use "politically correct" phrases. He said, "you are devils and you are going to hell". Dr. Robert Willner died under mysterious circumstances when he wrote something similar about the medical industry !

MOST OF THE research ever done on cancer is worthless.

A book which summarizes the state of affairs in cancer research says it as follows:

(Emphasis and bracketed comments by author)

MORE THAN 500 000 North Americans die of cancer every year. Yet while billions of dollars have been spent on research over the course of forty years we still have no effective treatments for the vast majority of advanced malignancies. Why are we losing the war on cancer? In his new book "The Immortal Cell, Why Cancer Research Fails", Dr. Gerald B. Dermer a dedicated cancer researcher provides a clear accurate and startling account of perhaps the biggest blunder in the history of science and medicine.

SCIENTISTS DEPEND on cells growing in petri dishes in their laboratories to give them information on human diseases. These petri dish cells, called cell lines, serve as models for human cancer cells. Cell lines are cultures of cells that are derived from tumors or normal tissue. But unlike any real tissue, normal or cancerous, these cells are immortal - they can grow for ever on the bottoms of petri dishes. And it is these manmade - creations that have become the favorite cancer model in the field of research laboratories throughout the world. But what if these immortal cells have been providing misleading, or worse, completely incorrect information leading scientists in the wrong direction?

THE IMMORTAL CELL tells an alarming story of unsound science and the pressures that lead scientists to do unsound work. It carefully details how researchers have squandered time, money, and lives in pursuing an enemy of their own making. It lets you in on what is really going on in the war against cancer.

DR. GERALD B. DERMER received his B.A. in biophysics, M.A. in genetics, and Ph.D. in cell biology from the University of California at Los Angeles. After two years of postdoctoral research in biochemistry at the University Lund in Sweden Dr. Dermer returned to Los Angeles and the Pathology Department of the Hospital of the Good Samaritan. There he began his research on human cancer, joining the faculty of the University of Southern California School of Medicine.

AFTER TWELVE SUCCESSFUL years in clinical and basic research, Dr. Dermer moved to the University of North Carolina School of Medicine, where he continued laboratory research for three more years. For the past ten years. Dr. Dermer has pursued his interests in cancer, pathology, and biotechnology as an independent consultant and writer.

THIS RESEARCHER carefully proves that the cancer treatments are based on false research! He has proved what many critics have suspected for decades. The mechanisms of cancer have already been discovered by hundreds of dedicated, brilliant researchers, from many different countries. The solutions (and there are dozens) have also been discovered.

RESEARCHERS WHO DARE to propose real solutions are viciously attacked by the pharmaceutical/medical/industrial complex. Many lose their careers, lives and enthusiasm. The heavily censored medical industry press, and the new world order media, ensure that the real solutions never reach the public.

FUNDING for research is dictated by the money forces of the world, who hold the purse strings of mammon.

THE FOUNDATION of the devilish cancer industry is based on false knowledge of causes, false knowledge of the mechanisms, and almost useless, severely destructive, outrageously expensive, cut/burn/poison treatments.

THE INDUSTRY IS SO fiendish that only Satan could have perpetrated such a devastating deception.

AIDS:

The hype and hysteria around AIDS is mysterious until the true agenda is known. It then becomes clear that it is nothing but another

"SYSTEMIC ATTEMPT TO create grievances in order to exploit them".

THE PRINCIPLE MECHANISM WHEREBY CONTROL, in a ratchet like movement, is reeled in from the masses to the authorities, is to create a problem, elicit cries for control from the people, and then place draconian control in place to de-power the masses.

THIS BOOK DOES NOT INTEND to deal with the political topic of world dominion, but public health is a prime target of the Satanic forces engaged in this process. The pharmaceutical/medical/industrial complex is the major co-ordinator of the plan in the health spectrum of human affairs.

NOT MANY PEOPLE die from AIDS. Compared to, say malaria, it is insignificant.

YET IT HAS BEEN PROMOTED to a hysterical subject, compliments of the media and the pharmaceutical/medical/industrial complex.

SEX AND HIV do not cause AIDS. It is caused by immune breakdown as a result of pharmaceutical medicines, environmental chemical/electropollution exposure, malnutrition, parasites (foreign protein) and narcotic abuse. (All these causes are big money spinners for the mammonites).

BUT, true to the Satanic sciences, A "big bad virus" and a "reckless" lifestyle are invented as culprits. "Blame the victim" and the "bad god" strategies at work again.

The brilliant researcher (Dr. Peter Duesberg), who was brave enough to expose the AIDS deception, was ostracized from the science community as well as from his career, and blacklisted, internationally, for his honesty. A summary says most of it:

(Emphasis and bracketed comments by author).

IN 1993, Dr. Willner stunned Spain by inoculating himself with the blood of Pedro Tocino, an HIV positive hemophiliac. This demonstration of devotion to the truth....was reported on the front page of the major newspapers. His appearance on Spain's most popular television show evoked a 4 to 1 response by the viewing audience in favor of his position against the "AIDS HYPOTHESIS ", yet this historic event was never mentioned in the U.S. press... Why?

ON OCTOBER 3, 1993, the London Times headline read, "African Aids 'a myth' ". Inside, across two pages, the headline screamed, "The Plague That Never Was", yet this story has not even been mentioned in the mainstream U.S. press...Why?

A MAJOR RESEARCH group in Australia has revealed that the **test for HIV is completely invalid, unreliable and riddled with false "positives." Measles, the flu, more than a hundred common infections and even a "flu shot" can render a person HIV positive.**

THIS STORY also appeared on the front page in banner headlines in the Sunday edition of the London Times, yet it too was never carried here in the United States...Why?

PEOPLE WHO TEST positive for HIV are in most cases completely normal and healthy. If like so many others, **they are placed on AZT they will be murdered by the AIDS it produces (AZT is the name of the drug used on AIDS patients) - thus the false and deadly prophecy is fulfilled! More than**

500 of the world's leading scientists have challenged the AIDS hypothesis -- they are being silenced, slandered and ignored...Why?

SATAN HAS EXCELLED himself with the AIDS deception. The diagnosis of HIV and AIDS is false (and the useless test kits earn billions of dollars), the stated mechanism of cause is false, the treatment is a deadly, slow poison (AZT) which makes millions of British pounds for the pharmaceutical/medical/industrial complex, the masses want "someone to do something", the medical industry look like heroes, and the gays are hysterical. Creating chaos and confusion as only Satan knows how!

READERS WHO ARE serious researchers can obtain masses of substantiating information from the well researched references in revisionist books.

WHEN ASKING ANY REGULAR "COOKIE CUTTER" doctor about AIDS, they will slavishly echo the dogma which Satan has conditioned them to perform, in Pavlov's dog style, namely that the patient got "infected with a big bad virus because of his/her promiscuity".

HEART DISEASE:
   Heart disease may not be as sensational as cancer and AIDS, but hundreds of millions of people on earth suffer from various forms of it, of which the most common is atherosclerosis (mainly blocked arteries).

CHRIST SAYS he provided abundant life, while Satan does exactly the opposite.

"THE THIEF COMETH NOT, **but for to steal, and to kill, and to destroy: I am come that they might have life, and that they might have it more abundantly.**" (John 10:10. (KJV)).

SOME STATISTICS WILL GIVE the reader an idea of the scope for Satan to "devour" and "rob and steal", in the heart disease "market".

HEART DISEASE EPIDEMIC IN THE UNITED STATES

Presently, (1993) More Than 7 Million Americans Have Been Diagnosed With Coronary Heart Disease.

EVERY YEAR 1.5 Million Americans Will Suffer a Heart Attack.

300,000 OF THESE Patients Will Die Suddenly - Before They Can Reach a Hospital or Can Receive Medical Attention.

MILLIONS OF AMERICANS Suffer Presently From Other Forms of Cardiovascular Diseases and Related Diseases :
    29 Million Americans Suffer From High Blood Pressure.
    8 Million Americans Suffer From Irregular Heartbeat.
    2.5 Million Americans Suffer From Cerebrovascular Diseases - (Atherosclerotic Deposits in the Brain Arteries).

THE HEALTH CARE COSTS (1993) FOR CARDIOVASCULAR DISEASES ARE SKYROCKETING

100 BILLION DOLLARS Are Spent in the United States on the Treatment of Cardiovascular Diseases Every Year - **$ 200,000 Every Minute.**

THE COSTS for Coronary Bypass Operations, the Most Frequent Surgical Treatment of Heart Disease in the United States, Amount to $10 Billion Every Year.

Survivors of Heart Attacks and Strokes Frequently Become Disabled and Live in Nursing Homes. The Costs for Nursing Homes in the United States Amount to Over **$60 Billion** Every Year. What an opportunity! And this is only in the USA in 1993. Imagine the size of the "market" in 1999.

Dr. Rath, and many other brilliant researchers, have discovered that more than 90% of all heart disease is caused by simple nutritional and lifestyle factors. The main cause is "sub-nutrition", meaning that the patient received too little, for their particular needs, over many years, of certain simple God-created vitamins and minerals.

These diseases can then be <u>reversed</u> within 120 days, by supplying the right nutrition. Very cheap and simple.

In advanced cases, intravenous EDTA chelation protocols can reverse the blocked arteries for 5% of the price of the medical industry route. (EDTA is the acronym for a substance used for clearing arteries and also accumulated brain toxins such as heavy metals).

High blood pressure is, in most cases, a simple imbalance between sodium and potassium. Patients can learn in less than an hour how to correct it themselves, via dietary reform .

Most, about 70%+, of blocked arteries are caused by long term deficiencies of antioxidants such as Vitamin C, as well as other nutrients like B6, B12 or the folic acid vitamin. In other words, some simple nutrient supplements can prevent and reverse this disease. If the food had not been perverted by the food industry, nutritional supplements would not even be required.

The standard medical industry treatment for high blood pressure is to prescribe diuretics (which loose and flush out minerals) and a low sodium (salt) diet. This is exactly the opposite of what is needed, namely, increased minerals salts and a high water table! Satan at 180 degree falsehood again. The medical industry exacerbate and amplifies the problem by doing exactly the opposite of what God created!

SATAN REPEATS the same formula for heart disease as with all the others: cause the disease with one or more arms of the team; then use the medical industry to treat the diseased people with outrageously expensive, semi-useless treatments, which cause more disease; use a third division to outlaw and eradicate any attempt at corrective, cheap, solutions; and finally, use a fourth division to "spin control" the relevant information.

THE MEDICAL AUTHORITIES in Britain (recently exposed, and with financially vested pharmaceutical interests) have spent the last year (1997/8) trying to get Vitamin B6 in Vitamin supplements restricted to 10mg dosages. To reverse heart disease, the patient needs 20mg per day! The very cause of heart disease via the mechanism of homocysteine, is a deficiency of Vitamin B6. (Homocysteine is a normal substance which accumulates and causes artery disease, due to vitamin deficiencies). Anesthetics are a major cause of strokes, up to months after the exposure to anesthetics.

THE PHARMACEUTICAL/MEDICAL/INDUSTRIAL complex is working through a global forum called Codex to have food supplements banned globally. Their international agencies: the World Health Organization and the UN, are right in there orchestrating it.

SATAN WILL NOT tolerate interference in his plan to destroy human health via the pharmaceutical/medical/industrial complex and the food industry. The foot soldiers of the Satanic movement are the doctors.

THE FOREGOING IS but a sampling of the "fruit" of the medical industry!

Does the accounting profession (the control group) bear this type of "fruit"?

The pharmaceutical/medical/industrial complex tree is undoubtedly Satanic.

OVERPOPULATION, ANOTHER LIE:

In order to render the practice of eugenics (population control) more palatable, and to set people up for genocide (killing of humans), Satan had to convince the world that there are too many people. The pharm-med-ind complex are enthusiastic supporters of this lie.

A 10-year-old child can disprove this lie by using a calculator and an Atlas. One can select a suitable geographic area such as Oregon, USA. By dividing the 6 billion humans on earth into the surface of the selected area, one will see that all the humans on earth can live comfortably in Oregon, leaving the rest of the earth vacant! Compared to Iceland and the Namib desert (where humans do very well, thank you), Oregon will be an improvement for most people.

"And God blessed Noah and his sons, and said unto them, Be fruitful, and multiply, and replenish the earth." (Genesis 9:1)

See what God says. Exactly the opposite of what Satan says!

Euthanasia and abortion, thus vindicated, become "generous contributions" by the people to the "population explosion" problem. Poverty, overcrowding and hunger are caused by the lust of the politicians to perform social engineering on masses of people.

Which just goes to prove, you can fool most of the people, all the time.

REFERENCES:
1. Galations 5:19-23. (KJV).
2. Matthew 7:15-20. (KJV).
3. Luke 17:2 (KJV).
4. Colborn, Theo. *Our Stolen Future.* (1997).
5. Chetley, Andrew. *Problem Drugs.* p 3 (1995)
6. Melville, Arabella. *Cured to death.* (1982)
7. Cain, Miriam. *Fight for Life.* (1995).
8. Proverbs 8:35-36 (KJV).
9. McTaggart, Lynne. *What Doctors Don't Tell You.* Chapter 3 (1996).
10. Psalm 106:37-41. (KJV).
11. Goodman, Rall, Nies and Taylor. *The Pharmacological Basis of Therapeutics.* Chapter 3 (1992).
12. Graedon, Joe and Teresa. *Deadly Drug Interactions.* (1995).
13. Mendelsohn, Dr. Robert S. *How to raise a healthy child in spite of you doctor.* (1984).
14. Contreras, Dr. Francisco. *Health in the 21st Century.* (1997).
15. Mendelsohn, Dr. Robert S. *Mal(e) Practice - how doctors manipulate women page 150-156.* (1982).
16. Exodus 1:16-17 (KJV).
17. Colgan, Dr. Michael. *Optimum Sports Nutrition. Page 249-253* (1993).
18. Wan Ho, Dr. Mae. *Genetic Engineering. Page 14* (1998)
19. McKenna, Dr. John. *Alternatives to Antibiotics.* (1996)
20. Cannon, Geoffrey. *Superbug.* (1995)
21. Miller, Neil Z . *Immunization – Theory vs reality.* (1996)
22. McTaggart, Lynne. *What Doctors Don't Tell You. Page 316* (1996).
23. British Medical Journal, *1995;310:489-91.*
24. 1 Peter 5:8 (KJV)
25. Miller, Neil Z . *Immunization – Theory vs reality. Page 29-30.* (1996)
26. Miller, Neil Z . *Immunization – Theory vs reality. Page 37.* (1996)
27. Matthew 6:24 (KJV).
28. Cannon, Geoffrey. *Superbug.* (1995)
29. Breggin. Dr. Peter. *Toxic Psychiatry, An all-out attack against the deception.....Page 378. .* (1993)
30. Chetley, Andrew. *Problem Drugs. p 204-209* (1995)
31. Contreras, Dr. Francisco. *Health in the 21st Century.* (1997).
32. Yiamouyiannis, Dr. John. *Aids.* (1995)

33. **McTaggart, Lynne.** *What Doctors Don't Tell You. (1996).*
34. **Carter, Dr. James P.** *Racketeering in medicine. (1992).*
35. **Laurence, Leslie and Weinhouse, Beth.** *Outrageous Practices. (1994)*
36. **Exodus 20:12. (KJV).**
37. **Moss, Dr. Ralph W.** *The Cancer Industry. Page VIII. (1996).*
38. **Willner, Dr. Robert E.** *The Cancer Solution. Page III (1994).*
39. **Matthew 23:33. (KJV).**
40. **CAFMR newsletter.** *(Spring 1996). www.pnc.com.au/~cafmr.*
41. **Deparrie, Paul & Pride, Mary.** *Unholy Sacrifices of the New Age. Page 122-125 (1988).*
42. **2 Timothy 3:13. (KJV).**
43. **Dermer, Dr. Gerald B.** *The Immortal Cell. (1994)*
44. **Moss, Dr. Ralph W.** *The Cancer Industry. (1996).*
45. **Goldberg, Burton.** *Cancer. (1997).*
46. **Epperson, Ralph A.** *The Unseen Hand. Page 37 Quoting Nesta Webster. (1985).*
47. **Willner, Dr. Robert E.** *Deadly Deception. Dust Cover. (1994).*
48. **John 10:10. (KJV)**
49. **Rath, Dr. Matthias.** *Eradicating heart Disease. Page 10-11. (1993).*
50. **Moore, Dr. Richard D.** *The High Blood Pressure Solution. (1993).*
51. **McCully, Dr. Kilmer S.** *The Homocysteine Revolution. (1997).*
52. **Goodman, Rall, Nies and Taylor.** *The Pharmacological Basis of Therapeutics. Page 405-414. (1992).*
53. **Pharmapact.** *(People's Health Alliance Rejecting Medical Authoritarianism And Conspiratorial Tyranny).* http://www.angelfire.com/biz/pharmapact/MAIN.html.
54. **Duesburg, Dr. Peter H.** *AIDS: Virus or drug induced? Contemporary Issues in Genetics and Evolution. Kluver academic puiblishers. (1996).*
55. **Stenton, Jean.** *Positively false: Exposing the Myth around HIV and AIDS. JB Tauris publishers. (1998).*
56. **www.virusmyth.co**

CHAPTER 7
SERIAL DECEPTION

"He that is not with me is against me; and he that gathereth not with me scattereth abroad." (Matthew 12:30)

CHRIST MAKES it quite clear in His discourse that there is no middle ground, one is either for Him or against Him.

"AND GOD SAID, Let us make man in our image, after our likeness:" (Genesis 1:26).

THE SCRIPTURAL PRINCIPLE OF FREEDOM OF CHOICE:
　　In the Bible evil is associated with the power of choice and could not exist apart from it. Only as beings capable of choice can one have moral responsibility; and this very power of choice makes evil not only possible but inevitable. It is a foregone conclusion that creatures who though made "in the image of God" (Genesis 1:26,27), are less than God (as any creation of God must be), will think thoughts and do deeds unworthy of God and thus evil by very definition.

THAT BEING the case why would God give mankind this exceedingly dangerous ability to choose? Why would God, who is only good, allow evil of any kind or even of the smallest degree in His universe? The answer of course, is obvious: God wanted to have a meaningful and loving relationship with mankind. <u>Without the ability to choose,</u> to love or to hate, to say yes or to say no, <u>it would be impossible for mankind to receive God's love and to love Him in return,</u> for real love must come from the heart. Nor could there be genuine praise and worship unless it were voluntary.

IT WOULD HARDLY BE GLORIFYING to God for robots who cannot choose to say or do otherwise to continually sing His praises.

THE TWO FUNDAMENTAL Scriptural principles that are dealt with in this chapter are:
   1. The fact that free will of choice is a Godly ordained property; and
   2. Interference in this God given freedom of choice is tantamount to turning against God.

THE EVIDENCE PRESENTED in this chapter will prove, from many different angles, and without any doubt, that the pharmaceutical/medical/industrial complex has developed local and global strategies to obstruct and destroy freedom of choice in matters of healing and all aspects remotely associated with health, disease and healing.

SATAN HAS of course calculated that when there are two choices, namely good and evil, and that if the good choice can be removed, then only the evil choice remains. With only one choice, the human is defenseless and automatically has to select the evil route. The pharmaceutical/medical/industrial complex achieves these devilish objectives by means of lies, deception, coercion, propaganda, advertising, manipulation, violence, pleading, planning, politics, philosophy, economics, education, media, social engineering, entertainment, TV, radio and movies.

THE ACADEMIC ANGLE:

For the political researcher, who prefers for these emotive issues to be coached in a more academic tone, the author recommends the following reading:

(Emphasis and bracketed comments by author)

THE BOOK ENTITLED "The Political Economy of Health" questions fundamentally the view that ill health and disease are misfortunes that just happen to people, and which scientific medicine is dedicated to combating. On the contrary, **it shows that ill-health is largely a product of the social and economic organisation** of society; that **medical practice and research** are strongly connected to their roles in maintaining and controlling a healthy labour force; and that the **medical field** provides a large and growing arena for the **accumulation of capital.**

LESLEY DOYAL AND IMOGEN PENNELL explore the changing patterns of health and illness and the evolution of medical practice in both Britain and the Third World. They include a detailed examination of the problems of **health as a welfare provision under capitalism**, consideration of the National Health Service in Britain, and a look at the part that **medical ideology plays in the oppression of women.**

THE BOOK PROVES THAT:

... the medical emphasis on cure (instead of preventive; author) is also of wider, though more indirect, economic significance. As we have seen, capitalist production is itself a cause of ill health in a variety of ways. As a consequence, any preventative medicine which was to be substantially effective, would need to interfere with the organization of the production process itself. Insofar as curative medicine appears to deny or at least to minimize the need for such preventative measures, it serves to protect existing economic interests.

IN OTHER WORDS, the forces which have the economic stronghold on the world, cause people to be sick, and then, to add insult to injury, make more money by treating the sick people instead of curing the disease, or preventing it in the first place.

PERSECUTION OF "REAL" HEALERS:

One of the most distressing horrors perpetrated by the medical industry powers is the vicious attacks on medical, and other healers who dare to employ "illegal" (in other words not sanctioned by the medical industry authorities) methods with which to heal patients. Literally thousands of caring, wise, informed, free thinking doctors have been hounded out of existence. Most have been murdered, maligned, decertified, raided, harassed via the legal and tax systems, deported, bankrupted and discouraged by the medical industry authorities. It is heart rending to read and hear their personal testimonies. Do innovative accountants (the control group of this book) attract such malicious treatment?

THEREFORE ALSO SAID the wisdom of God, I will send them prophets and apostles, and some of them they shall slay and <u>persecute</u>. (Luke 11:49. (KJV)).

CHRIST PREDICTED that people who bring the truth about salvation will be persecuted. It seems that bringing the truth about healing, results in the same punishment by the world at large.

SOME OF THE better researched episodes of persecution are summarized for the reader:

WHAT IS CANCELL, and why is it not available to the American public?

MANY PEOPLE SAW it on the Maury Povich Show. Could it really be true? Could a substance which thousands of people say has cured them of cancer be ignored by scientists and attacked by the FDA through the federal courts?

Could this substance, which has been produced and distributed since the 1940's, free of charge, which no one has ever made a penny on, be unavailable to anyone, even though it has been proven to be without side effects? This book asks those questions and presents the known evidence. The reader can decide, from the information in this book, what CanCell is, and what should be done with it. (author: CanCell is an electrochemical substance developed by a cancer researcher decades ago).

THIS BOOK simply asks that someone look into the evidence, test the substance scientifically, and answer those questions in an objective and responsible manner. Billions of dollars have been spent fighting cancer, and yet it is estimated that one in three Americans will contract some form of cancer in their lifetime.

Is it too much to ask that the evidence of laboratories, people who have taken CanCell, physicians, and specialists, even without a double-blind study, be taken seriously? Is it too much to ask that financial and political interests be put aside in the interest of helping humanity fight this insidious disease?

THE AUTHOR of the book is displaying the typical attitude of puzzlement which researchers experience when delving into the mysteries of the medical industry. People go through the same motions and emotions when first confronted with the disgusting practices of the pharmaceutical/medical/industrial complex. It normally exhibits the following sequence:

ASTONISHMENT (CAN I BELIEVE IT?), perplexed questioning (how can it be?), denial (it can't be!), indignation (how can they allow it?), naivete (the system will fix it), anger (look what they did to my mother), despair (the system is too big to challenge) and finally, inertia (I'll submit).

THESE SINCERE, albeit puzzled people, will be unable to grasp the enigma of evil in the medical industry, unless they view it through the looking glass of

Scripture, when it will become crystal clear that Satan cannot but invade the aspects of human health, which offer endless opportunities for "devouring" humans.

CANCELL, mentioned above, is a promising cancer healing substance which was eradicated by the medical industry.

ANOTHER FAMOUS "WITCH HUNT":
(Emphasis and bracketed comments by author)

THIS IS the extraordinary story of the **darker side** of "Science's search for the truth". It begins with the persecution of Jacques Benveniste, a highly respected French scientist whose career was **blighted** when he dared to expand the horizons of traditional science. His research provided an **explanation for one of the great mysteries of science**: the workings of homeopathy.

IN COLLABORATION with 12 other scientists, Benveniste performed experiments which he believes demonstrates that water can retain the "memory" of molecules it once contained. If this is true, then the laws of biochemistry would need to be completely rethought ...

YET THE LABORATORY of Jacques Benveniste was recently closed down by the French Institute for Medical research and he is now **deprived of any official means** to carry out his research ...

MASSIVE INTERNATIONAL PRESSURE was directed against Jacques Benveniste. Known or unbeknown to him, he had touched on one of God's most powerful sources of energy, namely water. Decades before him, Victor Schauberger, living in Austria, had discovered the same thing – he was also silenced, brainwashed and effectively murdered; the oppressive process only took longer than with Benveniste.

(Emphasis and bracketed comments by author)

"THEY CALL ME DERANGED. The hope is that they are right. It is of no greater or lesser import for another fool to wander the earth. But **if I am right and science is wrong - then may the Lord God have mercy on mankind**". *Victor Schauberger.*

WHAT BOTH VICTOR SCHAUBERGER AND JACQUES BENVENISTE were threatening to expose, wittingly or unwittingly, was one of God's free energy gifts, found in water, to humans. The only problem is that it would ruin the agenda of Satan's pharmaceutical/medical/ industrial complex, because it would create healing empowerment and independence, whilst the purpose of the Satanic pharmaceutical/medical/industrial complex is to disempower people and make them dependent.

THE AUTHOR HAS FOUND it useful, as a quick assessment, to use these criteria when evaluating any healing modality, namely: If a gift is from God it will create empowerment and independence of the world, whilst if it is from Satan it will create disempowerment and dependence on the world.

THE POWER and mysteries of water are severely understated in science. The author has studied the science of water – details which have only become available in the English language this decade. Water has characteristics and properties relating to life which are astounding. Only God could have created such an astonishing substance. When studying water, one is struck by one more proof of the majesty of God.

PERHAPS ENTHUSIASTIC SCRIPTURAL researchers can investigate the relevance of Scripture in the light of the enormous energetic power of water, with particular reference to:

"AND THERE ARE three that bear witness in earth, the Spirit, and the water, and the blood: and these three agree in one." (1 John 5:8. (KJV)).

AND, Christ speaking:
"He that believeth on me, as the scripture hath said, out of his belly shall flow rivers of living water." (John 7:38. (KJV)).

COULD it be that there are also literal meanings to these verses?

MOST TRUTHFUL RESEARCHERS are not even seen of or heard of by the masses. They are simply silenced before they are heard by the world. They also have houses to pay off, careers to nurture and children to educate. Most scientists can be silenced with a simple veiled threat that their promotion is in question if they dare to question the dogma.

ANOTHER DESPICABLE EXAMPLE OF PERSECUTION:
(Emphasis and bracketed comments by author)

THE EARTH SHAKING DISCOVERIES OF GASTON NAESSENS:
A MICROSCOPE that allows practitioners to view living matter at degrees of resolution **far greater than state-of-the-art microscopes currently available.**

THE SOMATID, an ultramicroscopic sub-cellular living and reproducing entity, which many scientists believe is the **precursor of DNA** and which may be the building blocks of all terrestrial life.

THE SOMATID CYCLE - visible in the blood of every human – which, when properly interpreted, can **pre diagnose degenerative diseases by up to eighteen months.**

714-X, a compound that has restored **the perfect health** of 750 out of 1000 **cancer** victims and that has equally dramatic effects with **AIDS** patients.

THIS BRILLIANT SCIENTIST was first hounded out of France and then harassed endlessly by the Canadian medical industry. His discoveries could prevent hosts of diseases and save millions of people from excruciating death. He could ruin the medical industry almost single handedly – that is why he was particularly viciously persecuted.

THE MORE EFFECTIVE the treatment is, the more serious will be the persecution. That is one reason why witchcraft and voodoo are not banished by the medical industry. Beware the day an "alternative" modality is officially sanctioned and approved by the medical industry – it has probably been perverted or rendered harmful or ineffective in order to comply with the menacing hidden agenda of disease creation and robbery.

THE 4 VICTIMIZATION cases cited in the preceding paragraphs are but examples of what happens in France, the USA, Canada and Austria. The same process is taking place all over the world – the citizens of no country are protected from the pharmaceutical/ medical/ industrial complex web of intrigue.

IN THE SCHOOLS

Children are brainwashed into seeing the doctor as something to be revered. They are comforted by the brainwashed parents with phrases like: "don't worry sweetie, mommy will take you to the nice doctor who will fix the pain".

COMPULSORY SCREENING and forced vaccinations are routinely foisted on the innocent children. Most parents are not even aware of medical industry visits to the children while they are attending school or even worse, at nursery school.

THE HERBAL INDUSTRY

Humans have used God given herbs as medicines since the beginning of human history. The herbs are effective because God designed the herbs.

"AND BY THE river upon the bank thereof, on this side and on that side, shall grow all trees for meat, whose leaf shall not fade, neither shall the fruit thereof be consumed: it shall bring forth new fruit according to his months, because their waters they issued out of the sanctuary: and the fruit thereof shall be for meat, and the leaf thereof for medicine." (Ezekiel 47:12. (KJV)).

HERBS ARE under onslaught by the pharmaceutical/medical/industrial complex. Herbs have been targeted for genetic engineering to alter the chemical composition originally created by God.

OLD STYLE herbal medicines businesses and companies are being "force" bought by the pharmaceutical/medical/industrial complex giants, where the herbs are being reclassified as prescription drugs at astronomical prices, and are subsequently only obtainable via a "registered" doctor and "registered" pharmacist.

INTERNATIONAL BORDERS ARE BEING "HARMONIZED" so that old fashioned herbs, vitamins and minerals become illegal. The United Nations agencies are prime instigators of this sinister, hidden motive of the pharmaceutical/medical/industrial complex.

"ASTRO TURF" AND "TROJAN HORSE ORGANIZATIONS:

Vast amounts are expended by the pharmaceutical/medical/industrial complex in order to create, infiltrate and abuse normal organizations like the "cancer associations", "ADD (Attention Deficit Disorder) societies, "Natural products associations", "diabetes foundations" etc.

THERE ARE EXPENSIVE, multilingual websites and magazines of which the sole purpose is to malign and discredit all forms of natural, effective, alternative or "controversial" medicines and modalities. These propaganda machines are massive. They issue a deluge of false information, promoting medical industry treatments and discrediting natural healing modalities.

THE RESULT IS that misinformation and sales propaganda can be dispersed to trapped audiences, in the case of the associations (astro turf strategy). Alternatively, under false veils, "holistic" organizations are funded and infiltrated, then hijacked to serve the agenda of the pharmaceutical/medical/industrial complex (trojan horse strategy). The officials running these organizations are often so deceived that they become unwitting cohorts and accomplices. Greedy humans are easy to entice with something simple like money. But then, no human will detect the deception clearly - only God can protect one from the sinister wiles of Satan.

LITERATURE:

All positive literature which is based on natural healing will ONLY be found in the lay press. Positive literature has been totally eradicated from the "scientific religion" press and libraries, especially at medical industry faculties. However, the lay press contains both positive and negative literature, so that readers are suitably confused. In other words the medical industry literature is heavily censored and biased. By presenting this grand lie (by restricting freedom of choice), the student will never be exposed to the truth, and so, will believe the lie.

TO PARAPHRASE ADOLF HITLER: "The big lie is much easier to establish than the small lie". And Hitler certainly knew the lie.

ONE HISTORIAN HAS SUMMED it up as follows:
(Emphasis and bracketed comments by author)

"THE SCIENCE of anthropology has had to be falsified to a truly astonishing degree to prevent information of this kind being universally known and understood. Many of those sciences whose purpose it is to help man understand himself – anthropology, psychology, genetics, etc. – are in the same state of eclipse today as were astronomy and other sciences in the middle ages, and for the same reason: that their findings threaten the foundations of existing power structures, whether these be religious or political or financial.

THE WORLD HEALTH ORGANIZATION (WHO):
Readers who are unfamiliar with the agenda of the WHO are urged to read the Christian exposé by Donald S. McAlvaney, entitled:

THE GLOBAL SOCIALlSTS' ATTACK ON <u>MEDICAL FREEDOM</u>: THE WAR AGAINST ALTERNATE MEDICINE.

THE WHO HAS a specific agenda to implement the pharmaceutical/medical/industrial complex agenda of depriving people of their freedom of choice, perfectly in line with their superiors, the UN, who are aiming to implement global oppression for Satan.

THE "LISTING SYSTEM:
This insidious tool was hatched by the pharmaceutical/medical/industrial complex to put the screws on the vitamin supplement fraternity. It was first implemented in Norway and followed by Australia. The sinister plot of this system is better known as "raising the hurdles", in other words, once the victims accept the carrot - the system of benign health listing products, then authorities start raising the hurdles by insisting on "labeling requirements", manufacturing standards , formula restrictions and health claims. Soon the small manufacturer cannot meet the raised hurdles and succumbs to bankruptcy or sell-out to a pharmaceutical/medical/industrial complex member.

MEDICAL AID OR HEALTH INSURANCE:

The medical insurance system suffers from two vulnerabilities for manipulation, namely an economic one as well as a personal one.

ECONOMICALLY, the medical aid derives fees based on turnover. Therefore, the higher fees and turnover becomes, the higher the income of the medical aid becomes. Therefore skyrocketing costs are welcomed by the administrators.

THE SENIOR OFFICIALS are also rewarded for including certain treatments and medicines in their "approved schedules". The pharmaceutical/medical/industrial complex thus places pressure on the medical aid society in order to exclude/include dictates in their policies. Should they "buck" the system, the medical aid society may be ostracized from the national "gang" and lose prominence, and to add to the punishment, the senior officials will loose their incentive "break away" freebie holidays and other personal gifts.

MINDSET:
The reader is probably inclined to react to these facts with the standard human response of disbelief. The way to remedy the disbelief is to perform an in depth investigation, like the author has done, and "see for oneself".

THE PARAMEDICALS:
Sub – species of the medical industry are divided into suitably controllable groups such as, nursing services, ambulance services, dietetics, physiotherapy, psychology, psychiatry, occupational therapy, dentistry, pathology and many more.

THESE ARE LIKE THE "TEMPLE PROSTITUTES" mentioned earlier in the book. The connotation is not sexual, but means the performance of evil tasks for reward. They are severely beholden to the medical industry, and ultimately the pharmaceutical/ medical/ industrial complex. All of these prostitute groups have "national associations" who are under the whiplash of the pharmaceutical/medical/industrial complex. None of the organizations, or the individuals belonging to the groups dare step out of line, for fear of reprisal or being "disciplined".

A TYPICAL STRANGLEHOLD is evident from the official "Position Statement" of the American Dietetic Association. All the temple prostitutes have similar "position statements".
(Emphasis and bracketed comments by author)

POSITION STATEMENT

"It is the position statement of **the American Dietetic Association** that the best nutritional strategy for promoting **optimal health** and **reducing the risk of chronic disease** is to obtain adequate nutrients from a **wide variety of foods**. Vitamins and mineral supplementation is **appropriate** when **well-accepted, peer-reviewed, scientific evidence** shows safety and effectiveness".

THIS RECIPE for disaster is forced on to all the gullible students and members of the sub-specie organization.

WHEN ANALYZING the position statement one sees the hidden agenda distinctly.

"OPTIMAL" health is what everyone desires. TRUE.
"Reducing risk" is what everyone desires. TRUE.
"...wide variety of foods.." TRUE, if from organic sources; FALSE if from the food industry sources.
"appropriate". LIE.
"well-accepted, peer-reviewed, scientific evidence". BLATANT LIE AND DECEPTION. The contrary is true.

SATAN'S WELL KNOWN METHOD, namely to mix the lie and the truth in order to deceive, is blatantly clear here.

Attempting to deceive Christ, Satan says: "**If thou be the Son of God, command that these stones be made bread. But he answered and said,** (and Christ answers): **It is written, Man shall not live by bread alone, but by every word that proceedeth out of the mouth of God.**" (Matthew 4:3-4. (KJV)).

SATAN FIRST STATES THE TRUTH, then presents the lie, just like the pharmaceutical/ medical/industrial complex. (If/Then????? Arguments). The *if* is normally true, and the "then" follows with the deceptive statement.

LEGISLATION:
All the world is party to the pharmaceutical/medical/industrial complex deception. Politicians are in their positions of power because someone sponsored and voted them into those positions. They are beholden to their sponsors for their political survival. The most powerful lobby in the world is the pharmaceutical/medical/industrial complex. They can enact any self-serving legislation they want to, even like insisting on banning Vitamin B6 in Britain, which would result in a massive increase in heart disease from homocysteine, as explained in chapter 6.

"NOW WHEN THEY WERE GOING, **behold, some of the watch came into the city, and shewed unto the chief priests all the things that were done. And when they were assembled with the elders, and had taken counsel, they gave large money unto the soldiers.**" (Matthew 28:11-12. (KJV)).

NOTHING HAS CHANGED, the church, the politicians and the rank-and-file are in on the act, conspiring as usual.

HOLOCAUST HALL OF FAME:
The pharmaceutical/medical/industrial complex have banned so many healing discoveries that a video compilation has been made to list them all. The title of the video is "The holocaust hall of fame".

FINALLY:

The pharmaceutical/medical/industrial complex have eradicated the major portion of the freedom of choice, in matters of health, from humans on earth.

MAY GOD HAVE mercy on them.

REFERENCES:
1. Mattew 12:30. (KJV).
2. Genesis 1:26. (KJV).
3. Hunt, Dave. *In Defense Of the Faith. Page 204-205 (1996).*
4. Doyal, Lesley & Pennell, Imogen. *The Political Economy of Health. (1979).*
5. Doyal, Lesley & Pennell, Imogen. *The Political Economy of Health. Page 37. (1979).*
6. Luke 11:49. (KJV).
7. Trull, Louise B. *The CanCell Controversy. (1993).*
8. Schiff, Michel. *The Memory of Water. (1994).*
9. Alexanderson, Olof. *Living Water. Victor Schauberger and the secrets of Natural Energy. Page 17. (1997).*
10. 1 John 5:8. (KJV).
11. John 7:38. (KJV).
12. Bird, Christopher. *The Persecution and Trial of Gaston Naessens. (1990).*
13. Ezekiel 47:12. (KJV).
14. IAHF. *International Advocates For Health Freedom.* http://www.iahf.com. (1998)
15. McAlvany, Donald S. *The McAlvany Intelligence Advisor. (November 1997).*
16. Journal of the American Dietetics Association. *Position Statement. Vol. 96 no. 1. (1996).*
17. Matthew 4:3-4. (KJV).
18. Matthew 28:11-12. (KJV).
19. Simpson, William Gayley. *Which Way Western Man? Page 699-713. (1978).*
20. The Life extension Foundation at: http://www.lef.org
21. Benson, Ivor. *The Zionist Factor. Page 137. (1986)*

CHAPTER 8
SINISTER SNIPPETS

"Beware lest any <u>man spoil you through philosophy</u> and vain deceit, after the <u>tradition of men</u>, after the rudiments of the world, and <u>not after Christ</u>." (Colossians 2:8)

"Prove all things; hold fast that which is good. <u>Abstain from all appearance of evil.</u>" (1 Thessalonians 5:21-22)

"The heart is deceitful above all things, <u>and desperately wicked</u>: who can know it? I the LORD search the heart, I try the reins, even to give every man according to his ways, and according to the fruit of his doings."
  (Jeremiah 17:9-10)

In order to understand the false philosophy underlying the medical industry, it is necessary to compare the way of Scripture with the way of "desperately wicked" man. The real cause of disease is Godlessness. Translated into worldly actions Godlessness leads to the destruction of humanity. The instruments of destruction are many, but physical health is destroyed mainly by malnutrition and poisoning.

Malnutrition is caused by the food industry. Poisoning is caused by the chemical industry, and their offshoot, the pharmaceutical/medical/industrial complex. In order to conceal the true perpetrators of the disease, the politicians (regulatory authorities) have to "invent" explanations for the chaotic conditions – they cannot reveal the real perpetrators, because the politicians will lose their power base if they do, in other words their bosses will end their careers.

JESUS WARNED the followers that the authorities and the church would all be participants in the destruction of truth.

BUT TAKE HEED TO YOURSELVES: for they shall deliver you up to councils; and in the synagogues ye shall be beaten: and ye shall be brought before rulers and kings for my sake, for a testimony against them. (Mark 13:9 (KJV)).

THE MOST DIABOLICAL strategy used by the medical industry to explain disease is the following repertoire:

1. BLAME THE VICTIM
In other words shift the focus of disease away from the true cause. This is best done by resorting to the "too" tactic. People are blamed for: "smoking, exercising, drinking, eating, sun-tanning, having sex, sleeping etc. "too much" or "too little". This tactic confuses humans beyond comprehension, because they will accept guilt for being "too" something or other.

ALSO COMMON IS to present some "mechanical" explanation to "soothsay" the concerned mind of the patient/victim; "blockages" of a pipe and "inflammation" of some tissue area are favorite waste bin diagnoses.

THE AUTHOR and his co-workers are astounded, and sometimes amused, at the bizarre explanations given to clients, by the doctors of the clients. Some of the more common ones are:

- "Your back spasms are caused by a hormonal imbalance in your brain".
  - "You have an iron deficiency which is going around town this time of year".
  - "Libido loss in your age group is genetic".
  - "A new virus is causing the loss of vision in your eye".
  - "At your age of around 45, 'chocolate cysts of the ovary' are normal"
  - "Your colon is misshapen and is causing the spastic colon".
  - "Your little sinus bones are malformed, thus causing sinusitis".
  - "A caesarian delivery will prevent a prolapsed uterus which is caused by a normal birth".

(It would be hilarious if less suffering were involved)

2. BLAME THE VICTIM'S PARENTS AND PREDECESSORS
The cause is thus said to be "genetic".

The victim is thus made to accept the disease as unchangeable, and will submit to medical industry treatment in docile acceptance of the inevitable. This is also where the standard medical industry curse is proclaimed, stating that "the patient will have to learn to live with it".

3. BLAME THE VICTIM'S MIND
The "psyche" of the victim is blamed for the disease. The victim is persuaded that the disease is "psychosomatic", implying that the mind of the victim caused the disease. At this point a brand new swarm of vultures can descend on the victim in the form of "mind experts" who will "correct" the "disease causing" mind. Enter the psychiatrists and psychologists, as deceived as their colleagues, the doctors. The difference between the two professions is that the psychiatrists

are trained doctors and thus apply a huge menu of mind destroying drugs to "correct" the victim's mind. The psychologists employ a counseling tactic known as "psychotherapy", invented by the likes of Freud and Jung.

4. BLAME THE EVER HANDY, EVIL AND MYSTERIOUS "GERM"

This is the stock-in-trade, ever useful scapegoat. So the nasty, spooky, invisible virus or "pathogen" can get the blame.

NOTE that the real causes are studiously avoided in the four arguments stated above. The reader need not fear that the doctor has become a little Satan, merely that the doctor has become an instrument of Satan. All four of the standard lies perpetrated on humans, as reasons for disease, are minor causes and cannot account for any of the epidemic patterns that are developing, while the genocidal plans of Satan are escalating to a frantic crescendo, worldwide.

THE PSYCHO-INDUSTRY:

When criticizing natural or non-medical industry healing, the medical industry critics are particularly fond of attacking the discoverer or founder of the modality, cleverly enlisting the help of their buddy church theologians, to prove that the modality is "occultic". This section of the book will now apply the same criteria, as used by the church, to the founders of the psychological industry.

THE REAL ARCHITECTS of the psychological system were few in number, recent in the history of the world, and have sold their strange mixture of Godless "pseudo scientific religion" and occultic philosophy to the world at large. Their ideas are in perfect harmony with misguided neo-Darwinian treachery and Newtonian physics.

THEIR THEORIES and techniques were devised by such acclaimed men as Freud, Jung, Rogers, Janov, Ellis, Adler, Berne, Fromm, Maslow, and others, none of whom embraced Christianity or developed a psychological system from the Word of God. Very few women had any input into the demonic hocus-pocus devised in the psychological philosophy.

THE TWO CHIEF propagators of the psychological system were Sigmund Freud and Carl Jung, both from Europe.

ACCORDING TO RON HUBBARD, Sigmund Freud was a cocaine addict.
Some scriptural researchers have detected the psychological lie, but most believers have been "seduced", "hook, line and sinker".

HUNT AND MCMAHON have the following to say:
(Emphasis and bracketed comments by author)

PSYCHOSEDUCTION

THE SEDUCTION **of Christianity** is definitely not confined to fringe elements. The **Freudian/Jungian myths** of psychic determinism and the unconscious have been so universally accepted that these unfounded assumptions now exert a major influence upon Christian thinking throughout the church. . . . As a **major vehicle of the seduction** that unites most of its elements, - psychology is **a Trojan horse** par excellence that has slipped past every barrier.

DAVE HUNT AND T A. MCMAHON: The Seduction of Christianity.

HERE IS THE TROJAN HORSE, mentioned in chapter 7, neighing and stamping around again, on a different terrain.

THE BRAVE PEOPLE who have done most of the exposing of psychoseduction, see it so:
(Emphasis and bracketed comments by author)

THE ROOTS OF RELIGIOUS ALTERNATIVES

FROM ITS VERY BEGINNING PSYCHOLOGICAL theories and methods of counseling **created doubt about Christianity**. Each great innovator of psychological theories sought an understanding about mankind **apart from the revealed Word of God**. Each created an **unbiblical system** to explain the nature of man and to bring about change.

MEN LIKE FREUD (1856-1939) and Carl Jung (1875-1961) **eroded confidence in Christianity** and established systems in **direct opposition to the Word of God! Occultism, atheism, and antagonism towards Christianity were disguised by psychological, scientific sounding names.**

SIGMUND FREUD REDUCED religious beliefs to illusions and called **religion "the obsessional neurosis of humanity."**

JUNG, an early follower of Freud, however, viewed all religions as collective mythologies. He did not believe they were real in essence, but that they could affect the human personality. While Freud viewed religion as the source of mental problems, Jung believed that religion was a solution. **Freud argued that religions are delusionary and therefore evil.** Jung, on the other hand contended that all **religions are imaginary** but good. <u>Both positions are anti-Christian</u>. One denies Christianity and the other mythologizes it.

RELIGIOUS BIAS COLORED the psychological systems of both Freud and Jung. They were not dealing with science, but with values, attitudes, and behavior. And because they were working in areas about which the Bible gives the authoritative Word of God, they were developing anti-biblical religions. **(exactly what the scientific religion camp did: author)**

JAY ADAMS SAYS: Because of the teaching of the Scriptures, one is forced to conclude that much of clinical and counseling psychology, as well as most of psychiatry, has been carried out without license from God and in autonomous **rebellion against Him**. This was inevitable because the **sovereign God of creation has been ignored.**

IN THAT WORD are "all things pertaining to life and godliness." By it the man of God "may be fully equipped for every good work." And it is that Word - and only that Word - that can tell a poor sinner how to love God with all of the heart, and mind, and how to love a neighbor with the same depth of concern that he exhibits toward himself.

PROFESSOR OF PSYCHIATRY and author Thomas Szasz contends, "The popular image of Freud as an enlightened, emancipated, irreligious person who, with the aid of psychoanalysis, 'discovered' that religion is a mental illness is pure fiction." He says, **"One of Freud's most powerful motives in life was the desire to inflict vengeance on Christianity** for it's traditional anti-Semitism".

FREUD USED scientific-sounding language to disguise his hostility towards religion. However, Szasz declares, "There is, in short, nothing scientific about Freud's hostility to established religion, though he tries hard to pretend that there is." Freud was not an objective observer of humanity, nor was he an objective observer of religion.

CARL JUNG REPUDIATED **Christianity** and became involved in **idolatry**. He renamed and replaced everything Christian and everything biblical with his own mythology of archetypes. And as he moved in his own sphere of idolatry, the archetypes took form and served him as familiar spirits. He even had his own **personal familiar spirit by the name of Philemon**. He also participated in the **occultic practice of necromancy**. Jung's teachings serve to mythologize Scripture and reduce the basic doctrines of the faith into **esoteric gnosticism**.

RATHER THAN OBJECTIVE observation and scientific discovery, Freud and Jung each turned his own experience into a new belief system and called it psychoanalysis. Freud attempted to destroy the spirituality of religion to illusion and neurosis.

JUNG ATTEMPTED **to debase the spirituality of man by presenting all religion as mythology** and fantasy. **Repudiating the God of the Bible**, both Freud and Jung led their followers in the quest **for alternative understandings** of mankind and **alternative solutions** to problems of living. They turned inward to their own limited imaginations and viewed their subjects from their **own anti-Christian subjectivity**.

FOUR MYTHS ABOUT PSYCHOLOGY:
   The first major myth is that psychotherapy (psychological counseling along with its theories and techniques) **is science rather than religion**. The supposition is that since psychotherapy is science, it is truthful and objective - simply another acceptable means of understanding and helping humanity. If the shepherds thought that psychotherapy might be a competing religion, they would surely guard their sheep.

THE SECOND MAJOR **myth** is that the best kind of counseling utilizes both psychology and the Bible. Those psychologists who are also Christians generally claim that they are more qualified to help people understand themselves and change, than persons untrained in psychology. They also believe that they are better able to help people than those persons who are trained in psychology but are not Christians. The ranks of this group have **multiplied rapidly** as Christians have adopted faith in the psychological way.

The third major **myth** is that people who are experiencing mental-emotional-behavioral problems **are mentally ill. They are supposedly psychologically sick and therefore** need psychological therapy. The common argument is that the doctor treats the body, the psychologist treats the mind and emotions, and the minister deals strictly with spiritual things. Ministers are then supposedly unqualified to help people suffering from serious problems of living, unless they are psychologically trained.

The fourth major **myth** is that psychotherapy has a high record of success. The myth is that professional psychological counseling produces greater results than other forms of help, such as self-help or that provided by family, friends or pastors. This promotes a further belief, that psychological counseling can be more effective in helping Christians than biblical counseling. The assumption is that because psychotherapists are trained in counseling, they are better able to serve the needs of Christians who need help with problems of living. And, that is one of the main reasons why so many Christians are training to become psychotherapists.

In examining the four major myths about the psychological way we will uncover a great deal of research, much of which lies **hidden in professional journals.**

Szasz further concludes that:
"It (psychology) is not merely a **religion** that pretends to be a science, it is actually a **fake religion** that seeks **to destroy true religion**".

He warns us of "the **implacable resolve of psychotherapy to rob religion of as much as it can,** and to **destroy what it cannot.**" Christopher Lasch, author of The Culture of Narcissism would probably agree since he says, "**Therapy constitutes an anti-religion.**" It is a fake religion that is "anti" the true religion of the Bible.

Another research psychiatrist has this to say about his own profession:

The techniques used by Western psychiatrists are, with few exceptions, on **exactly the same scientific plane as the techniques used by witch doctors.**

Does one hear accountants spewing this vitriolic type of criticism about their own profession? Proving once more that other secular professions are VERY different to the medical industry profession.

Psychological deception centers around the same principle as "scientific religion"; it is merely a subset of strategies to remove God and His Word from human knowledge. The author has noticed that when Satan perpetrates a real winner, it is normally <u>exactly</u> the opposite of the way God would have it.

So it is with the psychological industry. The mantra cry of the psychological industry rests on SELF ESTEEM AND SELF EMPOWERMENT. The way of Christ is exactly the opposite! namely:

"Then said **Jesus unto his disciples, If any man will come after me, <u>let him deny himself</u>, and take up his cross, and follow me. For whosoever will save his life shall lose it: and whosoever will lose his life for my sake shall find it."** (Matthew 16:24-25 (KJV)).

Denying yourself is exactly the opposite of self esteem!

The invention of the concept of "mental illness" is another massive fraud. The very name is an anomaly since one's mind is intangible, just as one's behavior or emotions are. How these intangibles get ill is beyond "scientific religion" to understand. According to Dr. Carl Pfeiffer, a pioneer in orthomolecular nutritional medicine, up to 90% of psychiatric conditions are simply due to malnutrition, and are easy to reverse.

ACCORDING TO SCRIPTURE, most of the aberrations of behavior are due to sin and/or demons, both of which can be solved with Scriptural healing processes.

ONE OF THE most demeaning aspects of psychiatry is the classification of sin as disease. The sinner is thus obviated of blame and responsibility because the doctor says the sinners are not sinning, they are "ill" and the mind-bending, brain destroying drugs are readily prescribed. Thus the patient is discouraged from seeking the cause of their disturbance.

(NOTE: EVEN THE ACTION OF "PRESCRIPTION" is derived from the occult which entailed consulting the astrological charts; "before, or pre-, making out the script").

THE NUMBER OF "MENTAL ILLNESSES" invented by the psychological industry have grown to more than 230. There is hardly a sin mentioned in the Bible that the psychological industry cannot classify and treat, in other words, they have developed a system to replace God and His Word, exactly what Satan, Jung, and the gang had in mind.

THE EVER WIDENING net of "mental disease" definitions, has ensured that the youth in England have a 10 times greater probability of receiving psychological treatment, than the probability of receiving a tertiary education! It simply means that the pharmaceutical/medical/industrial complex has achieved the goal of driving ten times more children insane, than the number of children educated by society.

PSYCHIATRIC DRUGS DAMAGE the brain of the victim, but are nevertheless routinely prescribed by psychiatrists with alacrity, and with a cavalier attitude. Children and old people are the hardest hit as victims of this form of chemical abuse. Permanent neurological (nerve) damage and suicide are common results of psychological drugs. All these drugs are designed to induce an "altered state of consciousness", the very state which renders humans most susceptible to demonic influence.

OF ALL THE diabolical characteristics of the medical industry dragon, the psychological industry must rank as the most evil. The author could not find one single positive aspect of this industry, other than in acute psychotic episodes. The whole psychological industry is a cesspool of demonic, lying, destructive, anti Scriptural and anti-God practices. The treacherous slime of deception which is cultivated in the psychological industry, has seeped in under the church doors, and has polluted the church practices to the point where "pastoral psychologists" are recognized officials in the church.

ALL SOLUTIONS for problems of the mind, psyche and spirit are found in Scripture. Any other solution is "another gospel", in other words, from Satan.

THIS CONCLUDES an overview of the Satanic psychological industry.

DETAILED STUDIES of the psychological abomination are available from "Psychoheresy Awareness Ministeries".

STEALING OFFICIAL BIBLICAL TITLES:
   The word "doctor" only appears once in the Bible. It is used to denote an expert of the law of the Bible, a cadre of officials also known as pharisees. These doctor's were teachers of Biblical law. The secular healing professionals were called "physicians", as was Luke, the disciple, who apparently performed this common occupation.

"THEN STOOD THERE UP one in the council, a Pharisee, named Gamaliel, a doctor of the law." (Acts 5:34 (KJV)).

"LUKE, the beloved physician, and Demas, greet you." (Colossians 4:14) (KJV)).

DOCTOR'S HAVE APPROPRIATED the title of "teachers of the law of God" for themselves! Instead of calling themselves physician (which they are), they want to be something else, something more religious.

THE PLAN of substituting the "scientific religion" for the real gospel is planned in the finest detail, even to the aspect of official titles.

THE SCOREBOARD SO FAR:
"Now the works of the flesh are manifest, which are these; Adultery, fornication, uncleanness, lasciviousness, Idolatry, witchcraft, hatred, variance, emulations, wrath, strife, seditions, heresies, Envying, murders, drunkenness, revelings, and such like: of the which I tell you before, as I have also told you in time past, that they which do such things shall not inherit the kingdom of God." (Galatians 5:19-21 (KJV)).

THE MEDICAL INDUSTRY scores 18 out of the 18 items, in order to "not inherit the kingdom of God", in others words the industry is leading to hell. From the Medical Tribune website of The New York Times, it is now also known that resident trainee doctors have experienced a high incidence of sexual harassment, sexual misconduct and noisy and lewd feasts.

BAYING HOUNDS INSIDE THE CHURCH:
One of the reasons which prompted the author to research the phenomena in this book was, years ago, when simply conducting innocuous trade in vitamin supplements, the Christian customers often inquired whether the

vitamins were not "occultic" medicines. Upon asking the Christian customers how they had arrived at that strange conclusion, (since vitamins had been invented by God), they invariably mentioned sermons and literature which had issued the warnings. Following up on that, the author inquired from the church leaders how they had arrived at that strange conclusion. The leaders would quote literature, not Scripture, but books and leaflets carrying dire warnings of all the devils awaiting people who stray from the "scientific " medicines of the western world. Following the trail further, to the origin of the literature, it would lead, mostly, to well meaning people simply echoing someone else. The propaganda trial ends at the massive propaganda machine of the pharmaceutical/medical/industrial complex, as discussed in earlier chapters.

As a result, one of the most distressing issues emanating from organized religion, is the all round condemnation of almost all "non medical" medicines. This status was achieved by means of multifactorial propaganda and indoctrination, by the pharmaceutical/medical/industrial complex, including all the mind-capturing strategies itemized in the first 7 chapters of this book.

The condemnation takes, on the one hand, the form of amateurish slogans deriding and branding all forms of "alternative" healing as "occultic". The other form of condemnation originates from highly "scientific religion" arguments by suitably qualified scientists and theologians, defending the "scientific religion". One can easily distinguish the treacherous arguments by looking for criticism of the medical industry in the presentation. The biased health propagandist will studiously avoid any criticism of the medical industry, or will make half hearted attempts to admit that, "at a squeeze", "maybe", "the medical industry", "just might", have a "few teeny-weeny, minor flaws".

There are 4 themes espoused by the critics of natural healing namely:
    -Defenders of the "scientific religion" faith. (they defend the pharmaceutical/medical/industrial complex.
    -Caretakers of the Christian faith. (mostly misguided Christians who genuinely want to defend their faith)

-Hollow chorus members and echoes. (echoing the dogma of the day)
-Attackers/deceivers/robbers/confusers hired by the medical industry (deliberate propaganda)

BOOK VENDORS who trade in Scripturally based books are well stocked with these devious attacks on all healing outside of the non - medical industry healing, better known as "alternate" medicines.

ONE OF THE most deceptive books, which serves as an insidious work of apologetics for the "scientific religion", and at the same time launches a detailed, academic "Scriptural" attack on almost all the non - medical healing modalities, was published under the title: "Encyclopedia of New Age Beliefs" (670 pages). The authors are described on the dust cover as follows:
(Emphasis and bracketed comments by author)

JOHN ANKERBERG HOSTS the nationally televised, award-winning "The John Ankerberg Show" He holds advanced degrees in **theology and philosophy** including two masters degrees and a doctorate. John Weldon has authored and coauthored numerous books dealing with contemporary issues. He has three masters degrees and two doctorates, one each in **comparative religion** and **contemporary religious movements.**

THE INDEX of the book does not even mention Freud or Darwin, two of the giants of new age philosophy. To make the lie credible, "real" occultic gurus, astrology, and shamanism are slated in the book. The greatest, and craftiest lie is the diabolical lie of omission, where the real evil is carefully omitted from the book, thus giving the omitted agents, especially "scientific religion", a silent nod of approval.

IF THE DECEPTION was perpetrated in good faith, (which the author has reason to doubt), the authors need major updating in their Scriptural knowledge.

C S Lewis, in his famous book "The Screwtape Letters", identified this type of crafty strategy, where the old devil teaches the student devil, that, by omission, some of the finest treachery can be perpetrated on humans.

Christ used a strong description for "learned" people in high positions who pervert the truth, namely:

"Ye serpents, ye generation of vipers, how can ye escape the damnation of hell?" Matthew 23:33 (KJV).

Ouch!

These perverted propagandists use various tactics to promote the hell bent medical industry. The arguments are usually biased, ignorant, bigoted, and produced by self styled experts.

A letter, sent to an indignant believer, who had been indoctrinated by the "baying hounds" in the medico/church pack, can serve to demonstrate the issue:

Dear beloved fellow believer: Re your fax on tachyons: Thank you for the fax, and the concern. These issues are of great importance to the Christian community "lest we are deceived".

Since most of the people in the world are NOT saved we find that most of the discoveries and innovations are from unsaved, secular sources. Since they are not from God are they then from Satan? Hardly. This includes textiles, cars, food and all man made innovations. Technological advances are particularly not made in the Christian community, because they have their eyes on the Kingdom of Christ and not on this world.

SHOULD you contemplate ANY item or idea of the world, you will be able to demonstrate in most cases that it is :
Used by unbelievers.
Developed by unbelievers.
Sold and manufactured by unbelievers.
Recommended by unbelievers.
Originated in an "occultic" country such as China.

DOES THIS MAKE THESE ITEMS "EVIL" to Christians? That would exclude almost all useful items and processes from Christian use. Many of the wonderful discoveries of the world were made by people, nations, and organisations with questionable affiliations, such as false gods. Thus God elects to whom His creation ("natural phenomena") is to be revealed. This principle is discussed in Romans 1, where the error of adoring the creation versus the Creator, is pointed out. The conclusion is that the creation and the natural mysteries it contains, are not for the exclusive use of either believers or unbelievers, but have been made available to all humans. Exclusivity is an issue when everlasting Life is at stake, and the choice is clearly made in the Word.

HOW SHOULD the Christian then discern when Satan has set a trap? In the "healing" industries we have to be alert to this issue, since we do not want healing at "any and all costs", and one of the costs can be alienation from God. Having meditated on these issues for the last 5 years, I have developed a model, which offers some comfort in the perilous journey through the health industry. The model distinguishes between <u>(A) Natural phenomena, (B) Evil Phenomena and (C) Technological advances,</u> made by humans. Examples would be (A) magnetism, properties of water, (B) seances, Satanism (C) computers, cellphones.

SCRIPTURE ISSUES WARNINGS against (B) for instance, divination and fraternising with familiar spirits. Any dubious pursuit or practice can thus be classified by the following means:
1. What does the Word say? - i.e. God's guidelines.
2. Is it a part of the creation? - as discovered by research.

3. Is it technology? - as made by humans.
4. What does the Holy Spirit say? - as disclosed to you personally.

REMEMBER that most of the creation is invisible to us ("things unseen"), and that all of creation consists of invisible components - (Hebrews 11:3). Using the scientific method - (another god) to discern, is futile, since that faith has spawned the evolution theory and many other abominations. You are left with the 4 items above as your discernment tools.

WHAT THE ITEM or practice is used or abused for, becomes irrelevant. An example, is that the use of black clothes is favored by Satanists, and that this preference does not render black clothes evil. Similarly, because the medical industry honors the serpent emblem, wings of Horus, and the staff of Asklepios, it does not render all medical treatments evil, (although most are). If a practitioner uses a device or procedure successfully, and uses bizarre explanations to rationalize the results, he is making the error, and the fault does not necessarily lie with the device or procedure. A primitive Christian, from a primitive country or background, may easily think that a hi-tech laser projection is "evil", because it seems supernatural in his framework of knowledge. Similarly a "modern" Christian who has been brainwashed by modern "science", will think that the memory characteristics of water is "spooky".

CHRISTIANS SEEM CONFUSED REGARDING matters of the occult. An example is the critic who maligns pendulums, (which he has never studied), but he is a daily patron of his favorite newspaper, which religiously prints the horoscope, as well as 5 columns of massage parlor ads - (prostitution). Similarly his wife warns of the dangers of oriental medicine, because it comes from a Taoist country (China), while she happily wears a silk blouse, made by slave labour, anointed in mystical factory rituals, and coming from the same China. All this while she is drinking Chinese tea and eating Chinese rice. Discernment indeed!

A GUIDELINE IS to employ the 4 points I mentioned above. Also, investigate a subject before drawing popular conclusions, or consult someone who has done their homework. There is a brand new cadre of Christian critics, who have become self styled experts on the occult dangers of alternative healing. They have no knowledge of healing, energy systems or the modalities they attack. Most of their rhetoric is gleaned from the propaganda, spewed by the medical/pharmaceutical industry, to protect the interests of the Illuminati. Unwittingly they have become cohorts of Satan in the battle to de-power people. <u>All</u> healing modalities may have spiritual elements lurking somewhere. Scripture, discernment and knowledge are the only solutions.

THIS DOCUMENT IS NOT a defense of tachyon usage. I have satisfied myself of the merits, as well as the potential dangers and would be loath to lead anyone astray. The research I have done at great cost, is extensive and the proof was sufficient to satisfy the 4 criteria stated above. How other practitioners want to regard these modalities, become irrelevant, since they do not always employ a Christian model as their discerning base.

BY ENGAGING IN SILLY ARGUMENTS, has already resulted the virulent development of over 3300 differing Christian denominations in this country (South Africa) alone. Lack of discernment in matters of the occult could cause even more.

THESE TIME CONSUMING and expensive un-learning efforts would be unnecessary, had the victims not been deceived in the first place. By listening to the "scientific religion" propaganda instead of the Word Of God, people will always be deceived.

BUT HOW COME MY DOCTOR DOESN'T KNOW ABOUT IT?
When presented with a truth outside the medical industry paradigm, the doctor will normally react with a robot-like, knee-jerk reaction by calling the truth "occultic", "mystic", "psychic", "new age" or "unscientific". The reaction is to be expected, because the truth is a challenge to, and in direct conflict with the medical industry "scientific religion".

The standard "cookie cutter", "scientific religion" doctor's are so spirit - and mind bound in dogma, indoctrination, demonization, red-tape, secular humanism, legalism, professionalism and occultism that ONLY the grace of God and the discernment of the Holy Spirit can help them "see" the truth and rid them of the bondage they have been seduced into.

SOME STRANGE PRACTICES IN SCRIPTURE

Before accepting condemnation by the medical industry, of any practice from without one's own paradigm, it would perhaps be a comfort to research some unusual (by today's standards) practices in Scripture.

"NOW THERE IS at Jerusalem by the sheep market a pool, which is called in the Hebrew tongue Bethesda, having five porches. In these lay a great multitude of impotent folk, of blind, halt, withered, waiting for the moving of the water. For an angel went down at a certain season into the pool, and troubled the water: whosoever then first after the troubling of the water stepped in was made whole of whatsoever disease he had." (John 5:2-4 (KJV)).

AN ANGEL, healing waters, Christ also showed up there, made whole? What would the "scientific religion" say about this? The medical control council would arrest the angel today for practicing "illegal medicine", and the church would condemn the practice as "occultic".

AND IF THE burnt sacrifice for his offering to the LORD *be* of fowls, then he shall bring his offering of turtledoves, or of young pigeons.

AND THE PRIEST shall bring it unto the altar, and wring off his head, and burn *it* on the altar; and the blood thereof shall be wrung out at the side of the altar: And he shall pluck away his crop with his feathers, and cast it beside the altar on the east part, by the place of the ashes: And he shall cleave it with the wings thereof, *but* shall not divide *it* asunder: and the priest shall burn it upon the altar, upon the wood that *is* upon the fire: it *is* a burnt sacrifice, an offering made by fire, of a sweet savour unto the LORD. (Leviticus 1:14-17(KJV)).

THIS PROCESS WAS PERFORMED to the delight of God. The "scientific religion" community would rate it "occult".

"AND THE TIRSHATHA **said unto them, that they should not eat of the most holy things, till there stood up a priest with Urim and Thummim.**" (Nehemiah 7:65 (KJV)).

URIM AND THUMMIN (mentioned several times in Scripture) were divining tools (yes/no answers) used by some priests to establish the will of God regarding specific matters. How would the "scientific religion" rate these devices? Occultic?

"AND HE SLEW *IT*; **and Moses took of the blood of it, and put** *it* **upon the tip of Aaron's right ear, and upon the thumb of his right hand, and upon the great toe of his right foot. And he brought Aaron's sons, and Moses put of the blood upon the tip of their right ear, and upon the thumbs of their right hands, and upon the great toes of their right feet: and Moses sprinkled the blood upon the altar round about.**" (Leviticus 8:23-24 (KJV)).

HERE, Moses is performing sacred rites, according to God's will.

WHAT EVER WOULD the keepers of the "scientific religion", in other words the professors, call this activity? The professors of theology (modern day pharisee's) would invent a suitably bland gnostic alibi, coached in correct politispeak, to keep the world at large happy, so that the audience may have their "ears tickled" and so that "the truth shall not reach them".

This argument does not set out to vindicate real occultic practices. What it does, is to illustrate that there are many enigmatic phenomena in the creation and in Scripture, which fall outside the field of materialistic knowledge. Because it falls outside one's paradigm, does not necessarily render it "occultic". The chauvinistic practice of brain washed, knee jerk, protectors of the medical industry, have relegated most God given, natural healing modalities to the forbidden trash heap of the always convenient occult thus placing Godly remedies outside the reach of modern humans.

CHRISTIAN DOCTOR'S?

Can one comprehend the anomaly of a Christian gangster, Christian paedophile, Christian devil or a Christian blasphemer? Perhaps, but the converted doctor will experience a "renewal of the mind" and get "out of Egypt" very soon after converting. The doctors face the same dilemma, in other words, once the doctors can see the truth, how do they ensure that they serve only one God, and not the god of "scientific religion"? It is an intricate issue which involves career, family and social issues. It is a matter in which only God can direct the convert.

THE NUTRITION LAWS OF SCRIPTURE:

Scripture , being the handbook for human conduct on the planet earth, has comprehensive rules concerning nutrition and hygiene. Leviticus 11 deals extensively with some of these rules. These "health tips" may not be crucial for salvation, but they certainly affect one's physical health.

CHRIST SAID:

"**It is written, Man shall not <u>live</u> by bread alone, but by <u>every word</u> that proceedeth out of the mouth of God.**" (Matthew 4:4-24 (KJV)).

By selectively picking at the Word of God, and "having one's ears tickled" by theologians who explain away the health and food dictates of Scripture, the perils of malnutrition and poisoning by the pharmaceutical/medical/industrial complex, become stark realities, unopposed by official doctrine.

It follows from the text above that one will die if one does not live by <u>every</u> word of God.

CAN HEALING OBSTRUCT SALVATION?

"**And a woman having an issue of blood twelve years, which had spent all her living upon physicians, neither could be healed of any, Came behind him, and touched the border of his garment: and immediately her issue of blood staunched. And Jesus said, Who touched me?**" (Luke 8:43-45 (KJV)).

THIS WOMAN WAS HEALED and saved by the power of Christ, in one moment! She had suffered from bleeding (probably menstrual) for 12 years (chronic) and had spent all her money on physicians (nothing much has changed in that industry), to no avail (as today). Had she lived today she would have been relieved of her uterus by means of a hysterectomy, and would not have embarked on the desperate search for healing, and would not have sought healing, perhaps missing Christ in the process.

WHAT ABOUT THE HEALER'S HISTORY?

Would one entrust one's health, or any other personal issue, to an ex murderer, wife snatcher, mass murderer, or say, a carpenter? These are some of the favorite servants in Scripture, in short order, King David, King Solomon, Paul and Jesus. This principle serves to illustrate that the past record of a saved person is of no consequence when it comes to serving God. Be careful of critics who insist on attacking a saved person, based on their history. It is a popular attack tactic used by the medical industry, against natural healers.

BEWARE, Satan can also heal.

OVERPOPULATION, ANOTHER LIE:

In order to render the practice of eugenics (population control) more palatable, and to set people up for genocide (killing of humans), Satan had to convince the world that there are too many people. The pharmaceutical/medical/industrial complex are enthusiastic supporters of this lie.

A 10 YEAR old child can disprove this lie by using a calculator and an Atlas. One can select a suitable geographic area such as Oregon, USA. By dividing the 6 billion humans on earth into the surface of the selected area, one will see that all the humans on earth can live comfortably in Oregon, leaving the rest of the earth vacant! Compared to Iceland and the Namib desert (where humans do very well, thank you), Oregon will be an improvement for most people.

AND GOD BLESSED Noah and his sons, and said unto them, Be fruitful, and multiply, and replenish the earth.(Genesis 9:1 (KJV)).

SEE WHAT GOD SAYS. Exactly the opposite of what Satan says!

EUTHANASIA AND ABORTION, thus vindicated, become "generous contributions" by the people to the "population explosion" problem.

POVERTY, overcrowding and hunger are caused by the lust of the politicians to perform social engineering on masses of people.

WHICH JUST GOES TO PROVE, you can fool most of the people, all the time.

WHITE COATS AND RED CROSSES:
   The medical industry has a preoccupation, and a centuries old identification with the use of white coats for doctor's and nurses, and the image of the red cross on hospitals, ambulances and related objects.

Even the shape of the red cross has to be of specific dimensions according to the international red cross society.

A superficial inquiry to the casual medical industry slave will elicit the response that the white is there to enable hygiene and the red cross is an internationally recognized symbol.

A more thorough inquiry reveals the real, and much more sinister, origin of these two occultic symbols.

The obvious question strikes one when working with disease, blood and human fluids, is that the users would prefer clothes which are easy to clean and have a stain resistant properties (for instance, the greens used by surgical staff make good sense, or the blue used by butchers).

White is the worst possible colour to use, unless of course it is used in a symbolic capacity, then it could be justified and make good sense. Chapter 3 illustrated the role of the demonised doctor as a replacement for the Saviour, who is symbolized by white. To supplant the Saviour, the doctor would need to fake the white light, even if it was impractical. The author contends that this is the only explanation for the bizarre use of white in such a messy occupation.

"For such *are* false apostles, **deceitful workers, transforming themselves into the apostles of Christ. And no marvel; for <u>Satan himself</u> is transformed into an <u>angel of light</u>. Therefore** *it is* **no great thing if <u>his ministers also be transformed</u> as the ministers of righteousness.**" (2 Corinthians 11:13-15 (KJV)).

Based on the evidence in this book, the doctor's are but "ministers" of Satan, also "transformed" into angels of "white light".

When researching the cross, one stands amazed at the subtlety and blatant occult worship, that Satan has installed worldwide by means of the cross.

To understand symbolism, one needs to compare the way by which God communicates with the world as opposed to any other way. To quote Gail Riplinger:

There are **two ways of communication:**
1.) direct and explicit (ie. The Word of God and it's doctrines).
2) indirect and implicit. (ie. symbols and rituals).

God uses the first method; Satan uses the second means.

Scripture forbids the use of images (in other words signs and symbols). This principle was illustrated in chapter 3.

All images, in any form, generate wave form frequencies which cause resonance in the target recipient. This knowledge is withheld from the scientific world at large, in order to influence defenseless humans by means of resonance. "Energy" has been declared a dirty word by the "church" which defends the "scientific religion", with the result that curious people are kept away from the truth.

Advanced practitioners in the occult make extensive use of signs and symbols, because they have known for millennia that energy can be mobilized via symbols.

It should be patently obvious to the inquirer that if the enemy of God loves something, it cannot be from God. All Satanists and occultists, as well as the fallen religions just love the cross in all it's manifest forms! Satan has tricked the masses again, with an artifact and lie.

Using a mere symbol to represent the cross of Golgotha is an abomination because it reduces the doctrine of Christ crucified to an image or gadget! Satan specializes in copying and/or demoting Jesus, especially by trivializing Calvary.

The original source of the cross is the mystic Tau of the Chaldeans and Egyptians – the true original form is the initial of the name of the god Tammuz (in Hebrew). From there it infiltrated all religions outside of Christianity.

Historian Will Durant observes:
(Emphasis and bracketed comments by author)

Paganism survived ... in the form of ancient rites and customs **condoned, or accepted and transformed**, by an often **indulgent Church**. An intimate and trustful worship of saints replaced the cult of pagan gods.... **Statues of Isis and Horus were renamed Mary and Jesus;** the Roman Lupercalia and the feast of purification of Isis became the Feast of the Nativity; **the Saturnalia were replaced by Christmas celebration** ... an ancient festival of the dead by All Souls Day, rededicated to Christian heroes; incense, lights, flowers, processions, vestments, hymns which had pleased the people in older cults were domesticated and cleansed in the ritual of the Church ... **soon people and priests would use the sign of the cross as a magic incantation to expel or drive away demons.**

The pharmaceutical/medical/industrial complex, being agents of Satan, have embraced the cross with enthusiasm. At the same time it could portray hospitals as places where life and refuge from woes may be sought, other than at the real cross of salvation.

Christ's message to the world is:

"**Come unto me, all ye that labour and are heavy laden, and I will give you rest.**" (Matthew 11:28 (KJV).

THE MEDICAL INDUSTRY has copied the essence of this message, as only Satan can. By disguising the doctor as an "angel of light" in a white coat, and holding up the red cross as the route to salvation, the medical industry has created a replacement for the real thing. To add insult to injury, this road leads to the destruction of health and the loss of everlasting life, as all Godless roads do. The medical industry performs a lead role in the game plan of Satan to destroy and control humanity.

REFERENCES:
1. Colossians 2:8 (KJV.
2. 1 Thessalonians 5:21-22 (KJV.
3. Matthew 12:30 (KJV.
4. Mark 13:9 (KJV).
5. **Carter, Dr. James P.** *Racketeering in Medicine. Page 190. (1992).*
6. **Bobgan, Dr. Martin and Deidre.** *Psychoheresy. Page 1. (1987).*
7. **Bobgan, Dr. Martin and Deidre.** *Psychoheresy. Page 12-15. (1987).*
8. **Bobgan, Dr. Martin and Deidre.** *Psychoheresy. Page 8-9. (1987).*
9. **Bobgan, Dr. Martin and Deidre.** *Psychoheresy. Page 19. (1987).* Thomas Szasz. The Myth of Psychotherapy. (Garden City: Anchor/Doubleday. 1978), p 25.& Christopher Lasch. The Culture of Narcissism. (New York: W W Norton & Company, Inc., 1979). p 13 34.
10. **Torrey, Dr. E. Fuller.** *The Mind Game. Page 8. (1972).*
11. Matthew 16:24-25 (KJV).
12. **Pfeiffer, Dr. Carl.** *Nutrition and Mental Illness. 8. (1987).*
13. **Breggin, Dr. Peter R.** *Toxic Psychiatry. (1993).*
14. Acts 5:34 (KJV).
15. Colossians 4:14 (KJV).
16. Galatians 5:19-21(KJV).
17. Matthew 23:33 (KJV).
18. Psychoheresy Awareness Ministeries. http://www.Psychoheresy.aware.org .

19. **Ankerberg, Dr. John and Weldon, Dr. John.** *Encyclopedia of New Age Beliefs. (1996)*
20. **John 5:2-4(KJV).**
21. **Leviticus 1:14-17(KJV).**
22. **Nehemiah 7:65(KJV).**
23. **Leviticus 8:23-24(KJV).**
24. **Matthew 4:4(KJV).**
25. **Luke 8:43-45(KJV).**
26. **Genesis 9:1(KJV).**
27. **Epperson, Ralph A.** *The Unseen Hand. Page 226. (1985).*
28. **2 Corinthians 11:13-15 (KJV).**
29. **Ripplinger, Gail A.** *New Age Bible Versions. Page 101. (1993).*
30. **Ash, David A.** *The New Science of the Spirit. Page 35. (1995).*
31. **Coats, Callum.** *Living Energies. Page 36. (1996).*
32. **Begich, Dr. Nick.** *Angels Don't Play this Haarp. (1995)*
33. **Hislop, Alexander.** *The Two Babylons. Page 197-205.(1959).*
34. **Hunt, Dave.** *Whatever happened to Heaven? Page 113. (1988). (Will Durant. The Story of civilization. Vol 1V The Age of Faith (Simon and Schnster. 1950), p 75.)*
35. **Matthew 11:28(KJV).**

CHAPTER 9
CONTROL AT ALL COSTS

The world of health and medicines is now so controlled, that very few population groups have even a vestige of self-determination, or freedom of choice where matters of health are concerned. The pharm-med--ind web of intrigue has enmeshed the whole world in a stranglehold which is rapidly and relentlessly squeezing the last pockets of health out of humans.

THE PACE IS QUICKENING, and the assault on health is conducted on political, trade, economic, scientific, religious, educational, media and many hidden fronts. People in certain countries have offered more resistance than other, less fortunate groups. The battle in the USA is fierce, and the "wounded dragon" has been exposed and is now a raging demon, out in the open.

IN EUROPE, health in only three countries has not been totally obliterated, namely in Iceland, Holland and England. The onslaught is fierce and only God can protect the humans against orchestrated global movements like Codex and the international pharmaceutical/medical/industrial police force known variously as "medicines control authorities".

THIRD WORLD COUNTRIES are still permitted to use "traditional" medicines, but the pharmaceutical/medical/industrial complex has targeted the traditional medicines for analysis and patenting, eventually rendering the original users "illegal". This form of "ethno-piracy" is conducted on a global scale.

ONE OF THE most despicable marketing strategies employed in the third world by sellers of baby formula milk, is to entice the new mother with free formula milk until her milk dries up, at which stage she is then DEPENDENT on formula milk for her baby, at which point she then has to start paying for the milk. This is called "creative marketing" by the food industry.

EMPLOYING THE LEGAL SYSTEM, as a means of raising objections, is futile. A damaged patient faces a daunting obstacle course when enlisting the "justice" systems of the world to confront the medical industry.

THE DIAGRAM WHICH FOLLOWS, illustrates the obstacle maze which has been created by the medical industry in Britain.[1] Similar models exist worldwide.

THE INDIVIDUAL HAS ABSOLUTELY no chance of challenging these monstrous systems.

ONE DOCTOR (DR. MATTHIAS RATH) who has challenged the system, has laid charges of genocide against the perpetrators. His charges are spelt out in the Tribunal document in this chapter.[2]

REFERENCES
1. **Melville, Arabella.** *Cured to Death. Page 205. (1982).*
2. www.rath.nl

- THE BERLIN TRIBUNAL -

On September 17, 1998 a Public Tribunal was held in Berlin against the Pharma-Cartel, Helmut Kohl and other accomplices of this Cartel for planning, committing and assisting mass murder and crimes against humanity.

DR. MATTHIAS RATH, M.D. who led the breakthrough in the control of cardiovascular disease by vitamins, convened this Public Tribunal on the eve of the Codex Alimentarius meeting in this city.

THIS COMPLAINT WILL BE FORMALIZED and submitted to the International Court of Justice and other courts around the world. Patients and people around the world are encouraged to take similar legal action against the accused of this complaint in local, regional and national courts around the world.

STARTING SEPTEMBER 21, 1998 the full text of this complaint will be made available via the INTERNET at www.rath.nl - a web-site that is currently contacted by several thousand visitors every day.

PREAMBLE

THIS IS A PUBLIC TRIBUNAL, a formal complaint to the International Court of Justice and other courts as well as a direct appeal to the patients and people of the world to bring to justice the pharmaceutical corporations, their executives, accomplices and all those responsible for the greatest crimes ever committed in the course of human history.

HUNDREDS OF MILLIONS of people continue to die from heart attacks, strokes and other diseases that can be prevented and eliminated. This holocaust is neither the result of coincidence nor negligence. The pharmaceutical corporations have planned and executed this mass murder and genocide willfully and systematically to further expand a global drug market of over one trillion dollars annually.

Prevention and eradication of any disease significantly reduces or totally eliminates the sales of pharmaceutical drugs for this disease. Therefore, pharmaceutical corporations systematically obstruct and even fight the prevention and the eradication of diseases. More than 95% of the pharmaceutical drugs currently sold are without proven efficacy while the severe side-effects of these drugs have become the fourth leading cause of death in the industrialized world. Thus, pharmaceutical corporations also promote the occurrence of new diseases as the basis for their expanding global market of pharmaceutical drugs.

To commit these crimes, the pharmaceutical corporations use a maze of executors and accomplices in science, medicine, mass media and in politics. The governments of entire nations are infiltrated and run by lobbyists and executors of the pharmaceutical industry. The legislation of these nations is corrupted and abused to systematically continue the mass murder and genocide of millions of innocent patients and people.

Throughout the 20th century the pharmaceutical industry was built and organized with the goal to control the health care system of nations by systematically replacing natural, non-patentable therapies with patentable and therefore profitable synthetic drugs. The architects of the pharmaceutical industry were unscrupulous entrepreneurs and financiers who, from the very beginning of this industry, had defined the human body and the diseases it hosts as their marketplace.

As the result of the systematic take-over of the health care system by nationally and internationally operating pharmaceutical corporations billions of people in almost all countries of the United Nations have been paying trillions of dollars for pharmaceutical drugs that neither prevent diseases nor cure them. The governments, the economic and social sectors of all industrialized countries are currently held hostage by the ill-conceived and criminal practices of pharmaceutical corporations.

A PARTICULAR EXAMPLE is the Federal Republic of Germany, the leading export nation of such pharmaceutical products in the world. Throughout the 20th century, the German pharmaceutical corporations Hoechst, Bayer and BASF have determined the fate not only of that country but of the entire world. In an effort to control the global chemical and pharmaceutical markets, these corporations formed the IG Farben Cartel already at the beginning of this century, sponsored the rise of Hitler to power and were the driving economic force behind the Second World War and Hitler's effort to conquer the world. Hoechst, Bayer and BASF were the organizers of the giant industrial plant IG Auschwitz using as their forced labor camp the Concentration Camp Auschwitz, the largest crime site of human history.

AT THE 1947 Nuremberg Tribunal 24, of the managers of Hoechst, Bayer and BASF and other IG Farben executives were accused of the following crimes against humanity: planning and leading the war, mass murder, conducting criminal experiments on innocent inmates of concentration camps, grand theft and plundering, slavery and other crimes.

THE US LEAD prosecutor Telford Taylor said in the Nuremberg Tribunal against these IG Farben executives: "Not the Nazi lunatics but these accused are responsible for this war. And if they are not punished for these crimes the harm they will do to future generations is much greater than Hitler could ever have done if he were alive."

THE IG FARBEN CARTEL was dismantled and split by the Nuremberg Tribunal into the daughter companies Hoechst, Bayer and BASF. With the help of Nelson Rockefeller, their former business partner and US Undersecretary of State after the war, all convicted IG Farben managers were released from prison already in 1952 and reassumed positions in the highest levels of German industry.

THE PREDICTION of Nuremberg Tribunal prosecutor Taylor soon became true. In post-war Germany the positions of chairmen of Hoechst, Bayer and BASF were held by war-time IG Farben directors and former members of the Nazi party for over a quarter of a century after the second world war.

HOECHST, Bayer and BASF lost no time to build up other political leaders to serve their interests in post-war Germany. Between 1959 and 1969 Helmut Kohl worked for the "Verband der Chemischen Industrie"(Association of Chemical Industry), the largest lobby organization of 3 the chemical-pharmaceutical industry. This industry systematically promoted Helmut Kohl political career thereby continuing to instrumentalize the German government for their global expansion plans. And their investment paid out. Now, fifty years after the Nuremberg Tribunal split the criminal IG Farben Cartel into Hoechst, Bayer and BASF each of these three daughter companies is 20 times larger than the IG Farben empire ever was. Today, these IG Farben successors are the largest exporters of pharmaceutical products in the world, maintaining an industrial network over 120 countries of the world. For almost two decades, Helmut Kohl has been heading the German government.

DURING THIS TIME the government of Germany became the political spearhead of the global conquest of the pharmaceutical industry and of the worldwide genocide and mass murder committed on their behalf.

THE CRIMINAL ROLE of the pharmaceutical corporations and the German government becomes particularly evident by the effort to suppress one of the greatest advances in medicine, which will lead to the elimination of heart disease.

THE YEAR 1990 became a turning point in medicine world-wide. In that year Dr. Matthias Rath discovered that heart attacks and strokes are no diseases. Similar to scurvy, they are the direct result of long-term vitamin deficiencies and they are preventable and reversible. It was also discovered that animals get heart attacks because they manufacture their own vitamin C, thereby maintaining optimum stability of their artery walls. Moreover, daily supplementation of vitamins and other essential nutrients were clinically shown to halt the development of coronary artery disease and also reverse existing atherosclerotic deposits by inducing a natural healing process in the artery wall.

THUS, it became clear that cardiovascular disease, currently the number one cause of death in the industrialized world, would essentially become unknown in future generations of mankind.

THESE DISCOVERIES TRIGGERED AN ENTIRELY new and basic understanding of medicine and human health, Cellular Medicine. Human diseases develop at the level of cells and the most frequent cause of cellular malfunction is a chronic deficiency of vitamins and other cellular bioenergy molecules. On the basis of Cellular Medicine today's most common disease can be largely prevented and eliminated including high blood pressure, heart failure, irregular heartbeat, diabetic complications, osteoporosis and other health problems thus far considered incurable.

SINCE NATURAL REMEDIES - available to everyone - are the solution to these health problems, it became clear that the time it will take to eliminate all these diseases is dependent on one single factor alone: How fast can the information about this medical breakthrough be spread to millions of patients and billions of people inhabiting this planet.

THE DISCOVERY that vitamins and other essential nutrients are the answer to the most common health problems of our time marked not only a turning point in medicine but it immediately threatened the very existence of the pharmaceutical industry.

THE GLOBAL PHARMACEUTICAL market of cardiovascular drugs alone is in excess of several hundred million dollars every year and the single largest segment of the global drug market. In order to artificially stabilize their global pharmaceutical drug market the pharmaceutical corporations now formed an international Pharma-Cartel. This Pharma-Cartel organizes a global campaign to systematically obstruct, suppress the dissemination of the lifesaving information of this medical breakthrough and to publicly discredit the health benefits of vitamins and other natural remedies.

BETWEEN 1991 AND 1994 and as a direct reaction to Dr. Rath's discoveries, the Pharma-Cartel tried to make vitamins and other essential nutrients prescription drugs in the US, their single largest national market. The pretenses under which the Pharma-Cartel promoted their legislative plan, "consumer protection" from non-existing side-effects and "international harmonization" to adapt inadequately low daily nutritional recommendations, were false and deceptive. However the statistical facts uncovered the deception of the Pharma-Cartel and showed that in the last ten years no American had died from side 4 effects of vitamins and other essential nutrients. Supported by millions of Americans, US Congress unanimously passed the Dietary Supplement Health and Education Act of 1994, which secured unrestricted access to nutritional supplements.

AFTER THE LARGEST national market escaped the control of the Pharma-Cartel, it turned to the international political bodies and found refuge within the "Codex Alimentarius" Commission of the United Nations World Health Organization (WHO) and Food and Agricultural Organization (FAO).

SPEARHEADED by Helmut Kohl and the German government on behalf of the Pharma-Cartel this Codex Alimentarius Commission is currently preparing legislation to outlaw all health information regarding the preventive or therapeutic use of vitamins and other natural, non-patentable health products in all member countries of the United Nations. To hide the real purpose of these plans they are promoted under the pretense and deception of "consumer protection" and "international harmonization" of nutrients. According to the Pharma Cartel, these unethical recommendations should become binding law for all member countries of the United Nations in the immediate future.

THESE CRIMINAL ACTS by the Pharma-Cartel and their accomplices deliberately deprive hundreds of millions of people of optimum health care. The direct result of these actions is the continuous suffering and premature death of almost every human being living today. If this mass murder and genocide committed by and on behalf of the pharmaceutical corporations is not stopped immediately it will continue and threaten human health and life in future generations of mankind.

BECAUSE OF THE historic and worldwide dimension of these crimes a comprehensive effort involving all mankind is necessary to establish justice.

TO INITIATE THIS WORLD-WIDE EFFORT, a public tribunal was held in Berlin, Germany on September 17, 1998, the eve of the "Codex Alimentarius" Commission's meeting in this city. Moreover, a formal complaint is filed with the International Court of Justice in The Hague, Netherlands.

AT THE SAME TIME, the full text of this complaint was made public through the Internet and other means to people all over the world. Patients suffering from cardio-vascular disease or any other disease mentioned in this complaint are encouraged to start litigation in their local, regional and national courts against the pharmaceutical corporations and their accomplices responsible for having prevented the eradication of these diseases long ago.

PLAINTIFFS

DR. MATTHIAS RATH, M.D. is the plaintiff in this tribunal on behalf of the patients of the world and the people of all countries of the United Nations.

Dr. Rath is the scientist who led the medical breakthrough towards the control of cardiovascular disease.

DR. RATH'S scientific discoveries that heart attacks and strokes can be eliminated by natural means, directly triggered the formation of the international Pharma-Cartel and its unscrupulous effort for a global ban of life-saving information on the health benefits of vitamins and other natural therapies. It is therefore incumbent upon this scientist to take the world-wide lead in stopping the mass murder organized on behalf of the Pharma-Cartel and bringing to justice those individuals and corporations responsible.

THE ACCUSED

THE ACCUSED in this tribunal as well as in any local, regional or national litigation on this matter are the following individuals, corporations and other entities:

1. EXECUTIVES of Pharmaceutical Corporations and leaders of the international Pharma-Cartel:
   a) Hoechst AG, its CEO Jürgen Dormann and all executives personally
   b) BASF AG, its CEO Jürgen Strube and all executives personally 5
   c) Bayer AG, its CEO Manfred Schneider and all executives personally

2. EXECUTIVES of other pharmaceutical corporations
   a) Merck Inc., USA and all its executives personnaly
   b) Bristol Myers Squibb Inc., USA and all its executives
   c) Pfizer Inc., USA and all its executives
   d) Roche AG, Switzerland, and all its executives
   e) Glaxo/Wellcome Ltd., United Kingdom, and all its executives
   f) Rhone-Poulenc-Rhorer, France, and all its executives
   g) Norvatis, Norway, and all its executives Further executives of pharma-

ceutical corporations will be added to this complaint as the now starting world-wide investigations proceed.

3. THE POLITICAL executors and accomplices of the world-wide Pharma-Cartel

a) Lead executor: Helmut Kohl Between 1982 and 1998 Kohl abused the entire political system of the Federal Republic of Germany to organize and execute mass murder and other crimes against humanity on behalf of the Pharma-Cartel, both nationally and world-wide.

b) Executors and accomplices:

i) Horst Seehofer, currently German secretary of health

ii) Manfred Kanther, currently German secretary of internal affairs

iii) Günther Rexrodt, currently German secretary of economics

iv) The government of the Federal Republic of Germany

Further political executors and accomplices of the Pharma-Cartel will be added to this complaint as the now starting world-wide investigation proceeds.

4. OTHER INDIVIDUALS and organizations in the field of industry, finance, politics, the media, science and medicine who, in the course of the beginning comprehensive investigation will be identified of having directly or indirectly participated in or contributed to these crimes.

COMPETENCE OF THE COURTS

I. THIS COMPLAINT is formally filed with the International Court of Justice in The Hague, The Netherlands, for the following compelling reasons:

1. The International Court of Justice in the Hague has the competence for trials against humanity. In a similar way, the International Court of Justice conducted the International Tribunal on War Crimes Against former Yugoslavia and against individuals who had committed crimes against humanity. The mass murder, genocide and other crimes committed by and on behalf of the Pharma-Cartel surpass those committed by any war criminals by an order of magnitude.

2. The extraordinary magnitude of these crimes essentially affecting every human life on earth urges for international proceedings in addition to any legal action that may be taken at the local, regional or national level.

3. To organize these crimes, the Pharma-Cartel abuses bodies of the United Nations Organizations such as the World Health Organization (WHO), Food and Agricultural Organization (FAO) and the "Codex Alimentarius Commission" established under the auspices of these UN-Organizations. These efforts directly contradict and openly violate the purpose of these UN-Organizations that were created 6 to serve humanity and not to harm it. Therefore, the International Court of Justice has a moral, ethical and legal obligation and responsibility to initiate this case.

II. This document will serve as a legal basis for all governments and member countries of the United Nations to italic officially italic support the organization of this International Tribunal against the accused at the International Court of Justice, through the United Nations Organizations and through other ways and means. People around the world are encouraged to hold their political leaders responsible if their governments delay such support that would bring to an end the ongoing mass murder and world-wide genocide committed by the accused.

III. This document provides legal grounds for litigation against the accused at any local, regional or national court world-wide for:

1. patients who have been directly or indirectly harmed, disabled, mutilated or in any other way physically or mentally damaged by the accused.

2. relatives of deceased who lost their loved ones from heart attacks, strokes, heart failure or any other disease maintained and expanded by the accused.

3. individuals or organizations filing class action lawsuits against the accused.

4. health insurances, corporations, governments and other entities filing lawsuits against the accused for repayment of damages in the magnitude of hundreds of billions of dollars.

5. any other individual or organization interested in bringing to an end the mass murder systematically committed by the accused.

CRIMES AGAINST HUMANITY

THE DEFENDANTS ARE ACCUSED of the following crimes:
1. Willfully and systematically maintaining cardiovascular and other diseases, including high blood pressure, heart failure, diabetic complications and osteoporosis that are recognized to be preventable by natural means - thereby deliberately causing unnecessary suffering and premature death of hundreds of millions of people.
2. Systematically and deliberately preventing the eradication of cardiovascular and other diseases by obstructing and blocking the dissemination of life-saving information on the health benefits of vitamins and other natural remedies –thereby causing unnecessary suffering and premature death of hundreds of millions of people.
3. Deliberately and systematically expanding existing diseases and creating new diseases by manufacturing and marketing pharmaceutical drugs with known detrimental side-effects – thereby causing unnecessary suffering and premature death of hundreds of millions of people.
4. Systematically and willfully deceiving the public with false, misleading and fabricated information about causes and treatments of most common diseases by abusing science, medicine, media and governments - thereby causing unnecessary suffering and premature death of hundreds of millions of people.
5. Deliberately and systematically abusing the legislative and political system to pass laws, establish regulations and promote public measures with the purpose to expand the sales of ineffective, unsafe but lucrative pharmaceutical drugs thereby securing exorbitant gains for the pharmaceutical industry and causing unnecessary suffering and premature death of hundreds of millions of people.
6. Systematically and deliberately abusing the legislative and political system to pass laws, establish regulations and promote public measures with thepurpose to ban, obstruct, legally criminalize and publicly discredit and deter the use of safe and affordable vitamins and other natural remedies

recognized to effectively prevent and treat today's most common diseases – thereby deliberately causing unnecessary suffering and premature death of hundreds of millions of people.

7. Systematically and purposely plundering of health funds in the magnitude of trillions of dollars from individuals, corporations and governments around the world by requesting payment for ineffective and harmful therapies.

8. Deliberately and systematically conspiring to pass laws and make other unethical efforts to continue all these crimes on international level thereby instantly threatening the health and lives of hundreds of millions of people world-wide as well as billions of people in generations to come.

9. Purposely and systematically abusing the United Nations Organizations, the World Health Organization (WHO), the Food and Agricultural Organization (FAO) as well as the Codex Alimentarius Commission to cover-up this organized mass murder and genocide.

10. Deliberately abusing the United Nations Organization for Economic Cooperation and Development (OECD) to systematically organize censorship of the Internet, with the goal to block and ban dissemination of life-saving information on essential nutrients via this communication path and thereby depriving the people of the world from receiving life-saving health information via the Internet.

THEREFORE, the defendants are accused of having violated human rights and committed the following crimes against humanity as defined in the Geneva Convention of August 12, 1949:

1. Mass murder and genocide. The crime of genocide is fully applicable because the crimes committed by the accused affect the entire human race.
2. Conspiracy to commit mass murder and genocide.
3. Direct and public incitement to commit mass murder and genocide.
4. Attempt to commit mass murder and genocide.
5. Complicity in mass murder and genocide.
6. Willfully causing great suffering or serious injury to body or health.
7. Plundering and extensive appropriation of private and public property.

INTERNATIONAL TREATIES APPLICABLE FOR THIS TRIAL

The following international treaties and declarations are applicable for this case:

1. The United Nations Charter.
2. The Declaration of Human Rights of December 8, 1948.
3. The Geneva Convention on Human Rights of August 12, 1949.
4. The Convention on the Prevention and Punishment of the Crime of Genocide of January 12, 1951.
5. The Convention on Non-Applicability of Statutory Limitations to War Crimes and Crimes against Humanity of 1968.
6. The Principles of International Co-Operation in the Detection, Arrest Extradition and Punishment of Persons Guilty of War Crimes and Crimes Against Humanity of 1973.
7. In addition, the defendants are accused of having violated the Constitution as well as criminal and civil laws of their own countries.

EVIDENCE FOR THE CRIMES COMMITTED

THE EXISTENCE of the pharmaceutical industry is based on business with diseases.

THE PRIMARY INTEREST of this industry is in maintaining and expanding diseases, not their prevention or cure. Following is a list of compelling evidence for the most immediate crimes of which the defendants are accused. In the course of the ensuing global investigation against the accused the full scale of evidence will become visible.

1. THE FOLLOWING specific evidence is presented that pharmaceutical companies are responsible for deliberately maintaining existing diseases and creating new diseases in order to extend their global drug markets:

a) Side-effects from the consumption of registered pharmaceutical drugs, is the fourth leading cause of death, causing each year at least 8,000 deaths in Germany and over 100,000 deaths in the US.

b) Only for less than 5% of the registered pharmaceutical drugs and currently marketed, a therapeutic efficacy has been established. In Germany alone 24,000 drugs without any proven efficacy are still being sold and have to be paid for by health insurances and their subscribers.

c) Drugs approved and currently marketed for the most common diseases, target the temporary relief of symptoms of a disease while avoiding to treat the cause of this disease. Therefore the patient is harmed several-fold:

i) The pharmaceutical drugs given do not correct the actual cause of disease and therefore these diseases persist in patients.

ii) The pharmaceutical drugs given may temporarily relieve symptoms of diseases while they frequently worsen the actual cause of the disease. Examples for this scheme is the marketing of diuretics for heart failure, which also flush out vitamins thereby aggravating the heart pumping failure, as well as the use of cytostatic drugs, causing immune deficiency, thereby accelerating cancer progress.

iii) All synthetic pharmaceutical drugs have known detrimental side-effects to the human body causing organ damage and generating new diseases.

MOREOVER, the pharmaceutical drugs are synthetic substances which have to be detoxified by the body. Drug elimination pathways are purely understood and drug administration frequently intoxicates the body causing new diseases or death of the patient.

D) THE ACCUSED ARE FULLY aware that vitamins and other essential nutrients effectively prevent and treat cardiovascular disease and other common diseases. In order to prevent the eradication of all these diseases through adequate consumption of vitamins by patients and the general public, the accused established through accomplices in science and politics inadequately low daily recommendations for vitamins and other nutrients. In order to intimidate the public and create the false impression that "overdosing" of these natural substances could be possible, the accused deliberately titled their recommendations "daily allowances". Without any scientific or clinical basis, the German "Gesellschaft für Ernährung" a cover organization of the Pharma-Cartel, defines 75 mg of Vitamin C as a daily limit for people while clinical evidence calls for at least 230 mg per day. By purposely fixing these low recommendations and by discrediting and even criminalizing the recommendation of higher values, the accused take yet another step to purposely maintaining diseases and preventing their eradication.

E) The following evidence is presented that most common health problems are preventable by natural means and are, despite that fact, purposely and systematically maintained and expanded by the accused:

i) CORONARY HEART DISEASE: The primary cause of coronary artery disease and heart attacks is a structural weakening and impaired function of the artery wall which develops - similar to scurvy as the result of long-term deficiencies of vitamins and other essential nutrients. Pharmaceutical approaches to the prevention and treatment of cardiovascular disease deliberately ignore this cause and focus rather on the treatment of symptoms, such as the reduction of cholesterol production in the liver. While deliberately avoiding to cure the disease for which they are marketed, the detrimental side-effects of these pharmaceutical drugs cause new diseases. The worldwide death toll from cardiovascular disease as a result of these deliberate-actions is in excess of 12 million lives every year.

ii) HIGH BLOOD PRESSURE: The primary cause of high blood pressure is an increased tension of the artery wall from a deficiency of essential nutrients in the arterial smooth muscle cells leading to narrowing of the artery diameter and rise in blood pressure. Pharmaceutical approaches for the prevention and treatment of high blood pressure deliberately ignore this fact. Pharmaceutical drugs sold for the treatment of high blood pressure purposely focus on the treatment of symptoms: Beta blockers and calcium channel blockers reduce the heart rate or diuretics reduce the blood volume. While deliberately avoiding curing the disease for which they are marketed, these pharmaceutical drugs are known to have detrimental side effects and cause new diseases. World-wide several hundred million high blood pressure patients remain uncured as a-direct result of these actions by the accused and their death toll is rising daily.

iii) HEART FAILURE: The primary cause of heart failure is lack of vitamins, minerals, ubiquinone and other bioenergy carriers in millions of muscle cells of the heart. This results in impaired heart pumping and accumulation of water in the body. Pharmaceutical approaches for the treatment of heart failure deliberately ignore this fact and focus on symptoms. Diuretics marketed for the treatment of heart failure not only eliminate water accumulated in the body but also washes out vitamins, minerals and other water-soluble bioenergy carriers. Thus the pharmaceutical drugs marketed for heart failure actually worsen the disease and they are responsible for the extremely short life expectancy of heart failure patients once diuretic medication sets in.

While deliberately avoiding to cure the disease for which they are marketed, these pharmaceutical drugs are known to worsen the disease, cause premature deaths of heart failure patients and are the primary cause for the extremely unfavorable prognosis of this disease.

World-wide over hundred million heart failure patients remain uncured as a direct result of these actions by the accused and the death toll is rising daily.

iv) IRREGULAR HEARTBEAT: The primary cause of irregular heartbeat is lack of vitamins, minerals, ubiquinone and other bioenergy carriers in millions of electrical heart muscle cells. This results in impaired generation or conduction of the electrical impulses required for normal heartbeat. Pharmaceutical approaches for the treatment of irregular heartbeat deliberately ignore this fact and focus on symptoms instead. Anti-arrhythmic drugs marketed to treat arrhythmia are frequently responsible for actually worsening the irregularity of the heartbeat and causing heart arrest and premature death of patients. The author Thomas Moore documented in his book "Deadly Medicine" that one class of anti-arrhythmic drugs in the USA alone caused more deaths than the number of US casualties in the Vietnam War.

v) World-wide over hundred million patients with irregular heartbeat remain uncured as a direct result of these actions by the accused and their death toll is rising daily.

vi) In a similar way, cardiovascular complications of diabetes, osteoporosis and other common diseases are systematically maintained and expanded by marketing pharmaceuticals deliberately designed for false and misleading therapeutic targets by the accused.

F) The following drugs and category of drugs are manufactured and marketed by the accused deliberately despite of their known detrimental side-effects and thereby causing new diseases under false pretense to fight existing ones. The fact that these new diseases caused by side-effects of these drugs surface many years later is used as an additional cover for this deceptive scheme:

i) Cholesterol-lowering drugs, particularly statins and fibrates are mass-marketed under the pretense of preventing cardiovascular disease. These drugs are known to induce cancer already at doses currently administered to millions of patients world-wide.

ii) Aspirin is mass-marketed under the false pretense of preventing heart attacks and strokes, while long-term use of this drug is known to cause an increase of heart attacks, strokes as well as other diseases such as stomach ulcers and gastrointestinal bleeding.

iii) Calcium antagonists are mass-marketed under the false pretense of treating high blood pressure and preventing heart attacks, while long-term use of these drugs is known to cause an increase of heart attacks, strokes and other diseases.

iv) Estrogen and other hormone drugs are mass-marketed under the false pretense of preventing osteoporosis and heart disease, while long-term use of these drugs is known to cause cancer in more than 30% of the women taking these drugs. Particularly frequent forms of cancer caused by these drugs are hormone dependent cancers such as cancer of the breast and uterus.

2. IN ORDER TO commit these crimes the accused have established a comprehensive pattern of deception ranging from fraudulent diagnostic terms in medicine to organized media campaigns to manipulate public opinion. Following are examples:

a) The accused deliberately and systematically mystify the origin of disease by using Latin and Greek diagnostic terms as cover with the aim to not reveal the true cause of the most common diseases to patients. The following evidence is presented here:

i) The true cause of high blood pressure is masked by the cover term "Essential Hypertension" = "High blood pressure of unknown origin"

ii) The true cause of heart failure is masked by the cover term "Idiopathic Cardiomyopathy" = "Heart muscle disease of unknown origin"

iii) The true cause of irregular heart beat is masked by the cover term "Paroxysmal Arrhythmia" = "Irregular heart beat of unknown origin"

B) IN AN EFFORT TO manipulate public opinion about the true nature of pharmaceutical drugs, the accused have subsumed pharmaceutical drugs under the fraudulent and deceptive term "ethical drugs". The word "ethical" is hereby used as a synonym for "pharmaceutical" and "patentable". This maneuver automatically implies that vitamins and other non-patentable natural therapies are "unethical" and therefore undesirable.

c) IN EXECUTING THEIR CRIMES, the accused systematically and deliberately extend their existing pharmaceutical drug market by inventing new health conditions for which they recommend these drugs.

The following evidence is presented here:

i) Aspirin was developed as a headache and pain relieve pill and is now being mass-marketed and recommended by BAYER for long-term use even to healthy individuals for the alleged prevention and treatment of heart disease and other severe health conditions.

ii) In order to extend the global market of their antibiotic drugs, HOECHST in cooperation with other accused fabricated and spread the so-called "bacteria-theory" of heart attacks on a world-wide scale. Without any clinical evidence that chlamydia or other bacteria cause atherosclerosis or heart attacks these accused criminally promoted the general use of antibiotics even to healthy individuals with the false pretense of preventing heart attacks.

d) IN EXECUTING THEIR CRIMES, the accused promote the alleged benefits of their pharmaceutical drugs through expensive advertising campaigns to medical professionals and directly to the public. The following evidence is presented here:

i) Public relation campaigns for pharmaceuticals almost exclusively feature the alleged benefits of these pharmaceuticals while deliberately ignoring, down-playing the known detrimental side effects or hiding them in small print.

ii) In order to finance these expensive deception campaigns the pharmaceutical corporations use more than one third of their revenues for advertising and public relation campaigns. This is more than twice the amount the accused spend on research of new treatments. Moreover, during the last decade the budgets of the accused for these deceptive advertising campaigns increased more than ten-fold.

iii) Millions of patients are harmed several-fold: They overpay for pharmaceuticals that do not cure their diseases and they involuntarily and unknowingly finance the advertising campaign for their own and continued deception.

D) IN AN EFFORT TO manipulate public opinion in order to conduct their criminal activities the accused organize, establish and maintain cover organizations. The following evidence is provided:

i) The Pharma-Cartel has established so-called "nutrition associations" which it uses as a cover to define and publicize inadequately low daily recommendations for vitamins and other nutrients thereby deliberately and systematically maintaining and extending diseases.

ii) The accused establish so-called "consumer protection" agencies who are used to create public turmoil about fraudulently alleged side-effects of vitamins and other natural substances. On behalf of the Pharma-Cartel and under the pretense of "consumer protection" these cover organizations publicly demand to make vitamins and other essential nutrients prescription drugs and to outlaw dissemination of health information in connection with these natural remedies.

3. IN ORDER TO commit their crimes the accused systematically infiltrate and manipulate science, medicine, regulatory agencies and even the natural health industry. The following evidence is presented here:

a) In order to continue their crimes, the accused focus their scientific, medical research and clinical studies almost exclusively on patentable synthetic substances and pharmaceutical drugs. Medical research is not performed with the primary object to find the most effective, safest and most affordable treatment for a disease, but with the object to identify the largest disease markets and to achieve the highest gains in that market for the drug manufacturer.

b) At the same time, the accused have deliberately and systematically avoided and omitted research and clinical studies with vitamins and other non-patentable natural substances. The first studies documenting health benefits for vitamins and other essential nutrients in the prevention of cardiovascular disease, diabetic complications as well as other common diseases were published over half a century ago. By systematically and deliberately neglecting and ignoring this information over decades the accused have willfully killed by omission to help millions of patients with heart disease, diabetes and other preventable diseases.

c) In order to systematically organize their crimes the accused infiltrated the medical profession, which previously had been applying almost exclusively natural therapies. These natural therapeutic approaches were systematically removed from the training programs at medical schools, purposely producing generations of doctors with little or no knowledge about the lifesaving health benefits of vitamins and other natural therapies. Simultaneously, therapeutic education at medical schools was reorganized, taken over by newly created departments of pharmacology and generations of doctors are leaving medical schools practically as a trained sales force for the Pharma-Cartel.

d) To systematically organize the expansion of their crime scheme the accused created an ever increasing number of synthetic substances to be marketed as pharmaceuticals. In order to accelerate the introduction of these new pharmaceuticals to the health market the accused systematically infiltrated the drug regulatory agencies and registration authorities of the governments. As a result most so-called experts of these approval committees are on the payroll of the Pharma-Cartel.

e) In order to undermine and neutralize resistance against new regulations from the health food industry and consumers, the Pharma-Cartel even infiltrates the nutritional supplement industry. The following evidence is provided:

In 1996 the accused Pharma-Cartel member Hoechst forged a strategic alliance with Rexall/Sundown, a Florida based nutritional supplement manufacturer. Rexall/Sundown, a publicly known cover organization for Organized Crime and the Genovese Crime Family, is now using its influence in the US nutrition and health food industry. The "Council for Responsible Nutrition (CRN)" and other associations of the health food industry are now accepting self imposed limitations on health claims in relation to vitamins and natural therapies, thereby undermining the Dietary Supplement Health and Education Act of 1994 and depleting patients of life-saving information.

4. To PROMOTE their criminal plans on a world-wide scale and to lend their crimes the cover of legitimacy, the accused abuse the legislative bodies on

national and international levels. They influence, manipulate and bribe politicians and systematically promote their own lobbyists into highest political positions and offices. Particularly evident is the influence of the accused on the government, the legislation and the administrative bodies of Germany. It is via the government of this country, Germany, that the Pharma-Cartel and its political executors are currently trying to extend and establish their criminal plans on a global scale by systematically abusing the United Nations Organizations.

a) Influencing and abusing legislation, the accused arbitrarily defined in their Arzneimittel-Gesetz (Drug Law) that Vitamin C pills over and above 500 mg are considered prescription drugs. This unethical law ignores the fact that most animals produce up to 20 grams of vitamin C, compared to the human body weight, in their own bodies – physiologically and for millions of years without any side-effects.

b) Despite the fact that this law has no scientific basis, its violation is defined by the accused as a crime and prosecuted by means of their access to administrative and law enforcement means.

c) The particularly malicious restriction of vitamin C by the accused has no medical or scientific basis, it rather serves the criminal plans of the Pharma-Cartel to further expand diseases. Vitamin C is one of the most important molecules for human health and life in general. By discrediting and criminalizing this very essence of human health, the accused deliberately and systematically impair the health as well as promote common diseases in millions of people as a basis for expanding their global drug sales.

d) This criminal legislation is now being further extended. Because a growing number of German citizens is obtaining their essential nutrients from abroad, a new law was introduced under the pretense of "consumer protection" that also prohibits and criminalizes the import of vitamin C pills above 500 mg - even from within the European Community.

e) Particularly aggravating is the fact that the main political executor of the Pharma-Cartel, the accused Helmut Kohl himself, initiated this law. On March 27, 1998 Kohl initiated the "Erstes Änderungsgesetz zum Medizinproduktegesetz" (First amendment to the Medical Product Law). As documented on the German government's Internet, this was only three days after the news about Dr. Rath's breakthrough discoveries and the clinical proof of natural reversal of coronary artery disease by vitamin supplementation aired on national German TV in the prime-time show Frontal of Zweites Deutsches

Fernsehen (ZDF). Thus, shortly after millions of people in Germany had learned for the first time that optimum vitamin C intake can prevent and effectively treat the most common disease, the accused Pharma-Cartel executor Helmut Kohl, initiates a federal law that obstructs and bans the implementation of this health measure. With full understanding of the consequences, the accused Helmut Kohl guarantees the continuation of cardiovascular disease and of ongoing sales for cardiovascular pharmaceuticals. With his acts, he deliberately and maliciously compromises the health and shortens the life of millions of people in Germany and beyond.

f) The accused Helmut Kohl has violated the Constitution of Germany, breached his oath of office to protect German citizens from harm as well as national and international criminal laws. He has personally harmed millions of people and bears personal responsibility for that crime.

g) A further aggravating fact is the context of the political career of the accused Helmut Kohl:

h) His constituency is Ludwigshafen, the same city where BASF, one of the principals of the Pharma-Cartel and also accused here, maintains its world headquarters.

ii) From 1959 to 1969 the accused was employed by the "Verband der Chemischen Industrie", the largest pharmaceutical-chemical lobby organization in Germany. The German Pharma-Cartel promoted Helmut Kohl's political career up to the head of state.

iii) Helmut Kohl's personal political mentor Dr. Riess was a war criminal in the Second World War. Dr. Riess owned and operated the "Oberslesische Gummiwerke" (Rubber plant Upper Silesia) only a few miles away from the concentration camp Auschwitz. He exploited thousands of innocent inmates from this concentration camp as forced labor. In 1971 Helmut Kohl rewarded his political mentor Dr. Riess with the highest honor of Germany, the Bundes-verdienstkreuz (Federal Cross of Merit). Details can be obtained from the books of Bernt Engelmann, the former President of the "Deutscher Schriftstellerverband" (German writers association).

h) Accused is the entire German government. This government, led by Helmut Kohl has systematically implemented the criminal plans of the Pharma-Cartel on national and international level. In the interest of this cartel it is continuing to abuse the United Nations and its organizations WHO, FAO, OECD, Codex Alimentarius as well as other international bodies. INDIVIDUAL CRIMINAL RESPONSIBILITY Because the accused, like those in the Nuremberg Tribunal, could seek refuge in a defense that they acted in their capacity as politicians or upon request of superiors, the following provisions have to be part of the tribunal proceedings: An accused who planned, instigated, ordered, committed or otherwise aided and abetted in the planning, preparation or execution of a crime referred to in this complaint, shall be individually responsible for the crime.

THE OFFICIAL POSITION of any accused person, whether as executive of a corporation, as Head of State or Government, as a responsible Government official or in any other public or private function shall not relieve such person of criminal responsibility nor mitigate punishment. The fact that any of the acts referred to in this complaint was committed by a subordinate does not relieve his superior of criminal responsibility if he knew or had reason to know that the subordinate was about to commit such acts or had done so. The fact that an accused person acted pursuant to an order of a government or of a superior shall not relieve him of criminal responsibility. The lead corporations of the Pharma-Cartel accused in this case are identical with the corporations accused in the Nuremberg Tribunal for the crimes committed in the second World War, namely Hoechst, Bayer and BASF. In the Nuremberg Tribunal the executives of these corporations tried to excuse themselves from any guilt by blaming the doctors who administered the drugs on their behalf. The deadly experiments conducted on concentration camp inmates with typhus vaccines on behalf of Bayer and Hoechst were blamed on the doctors applying these procedures. In fact, several medical doctors were sentenced to death in the Nuremberg Tribunal, while the responsible corporate executives of Hoechst and Bayer were released from prison. Any forthcoming trial has to take particular care that this line of defense by the accused corporations and executives is excluded from the beginning. Those responsible of the Pharma-Cartel, especially the executives of Hoechst, Bayer and BASF, as well as their political arm, Helmut Kohl, must be held to the full extent, personally responsible for those crimes against the human rights. This complaint is the starting point for a world-wide campaign against the crimes committed by the pharmaceutical companies and the Pharma-Cartel, as well as their accomplices in politics, media, science and medicine. Further individuals and organizations can at all times be included in a further complaint and can be prosecuted in an international tribunal as well in regional and national courts.

FINAL PLEAD

IF THE ACCUSED in this complaint are brought to justice, mankind has the opportunity to liberate itself from the most common diseases of the industrial world, including heart attacks, strokes, heart failure, complications of diabetes, osteoporosis and many others. Millions of lives will be saved and the quality of life as well as life expectancy will rise for this generation and generations to come. The redistribution of the wealth robbed by the accused will serve millions of people, and the economies of all countries of the United Nations. Health will become a human right not only for the industrialized world. The new funds available will also be used for the developing world for health education as well as preventive and primary health care measures. This will inevitably lead to an improved standard of living in these countries and to a decrease in the current gap between rich and poor countries. Obstruction of these efforts will inevitably continue these preventable diseases resulting in unnecessary suffering and death of millions of people.

CHAPTER 10
PARTING THOUGHTS

The reader must be wondering whether one can risk one's health by submitting one's body and spirit to the medical industry at all. Is there anything good in the medical industry?

THE AUTHOR GIVES it a qualified yes, with a strong reservation. Only submit to the medical industry as a last resort in times of acute crisis, for example mechanical accidents, poisoning or unconsciousness. The medical industry is normally appropriate in acute care (meaning crisis, short term, infrequent).

ANYONE WHO IS GIVEN to "doctor bashing" should spend a Friday nightshift in a busy trauma unit of a city hospital. That is where technology can reverse some of the devastation caused by mechanical damage to the human body – but that is not healing, it is mechanical repair work, and that is the triumph of modern medicine.

THERE ARE ALSO rare instances during a confinement where a baby's, or the mother's life may be saved by a doctor, again as a last resort. This is a fine line, because if the doctor arrives before the crisis does, the doctor will most likely create complications and precipitate a crisis.

PATHOLOGICAL (MEDICAL TEST) reports can provide useful information in respect of blood and other body-chemical profiles. Blood pressure and alkalinity are useful markers, but they are tests which the patients can learn to perform at home.

SOME CHRONIC CONDITIONS, such as insulin dependant diabetes, caused by (for instance) antibiotic damage, are life-dependant on insulin injections and the monitoring of blood sugar levels. These can both be done at home by the patient and do not require a doctor. In any case, the insulin is not a drug, since it is simply a copy of the body-identical, human insulin hormone. The medical industry would like to claim credit for insulin, but God made it, science only copied the real thing! Many insulin dependant diabetics have seen their diabetic condition reversed with the application of non-medical modalities.

MANY DOCTOR'S HAVE "CONVERTED" to natural healing, in spite of the medical industry, by their own determination. It is estimated that 1% of USA doctors have crossed the rubicon into natural healing. They find themselves on a massive curve of learning the new, and unlearning the lie, incurring a drop in income, as well as facing the ire of the medical industry establishment and their colleagues. These are brave individuals indeed.

ARE all doctors then demonised and agents of Satan? Considering the ritualization and reinforcement thereof in the medical industry systems, the doctor, unless released of the bondage of his oath, and cleansed by the blood of Christ, is still "in the spiritual Egypt", with all the timeless and diabolical implications associated with being cursed by God and Satan.

WHAT IF ONE has beloved friends or relatives who have been trapped inside the medical industry, as doctor's or paramedicals? Prayer, asking for the grace of God to give them deliverance and clarity of view, is the only solution that the author knows of. Reasoning with the trapped people is futile because they have been blinded and have been taught knee-jerk responses to all the arguments based on science, philosophy, reason and morals. If they have not been saved, one merely annoys them by advancing health arguments based on God's principles, Paradigm differences exist between saved healers and medical industry healers, making intelligible discussions almost impossible. The 7 most common pitfalls during any such discussion, are listed below:

MEDICAL PARADIGM PROBLEMS

SOME REASONS why natural healers and medical scientists have difficulties when attempting the sensible exchange of ideas.

1. THE EVOLUTION theory vs the creation approach. Medical scientists are trained in a setting which upholds the evolution theory, while most natural healers believe that nature was created by God. Tonsils, to a medical scientist, are for instance dispensable, while the natural healers would be repelled by the thought.

2. THE GERM theory (Pasteur) of disease vs the terrain (Claude Bernard and Antoine Béchamp) approach. The medical scientists insist that germs cause disease, whilst the natural school maintain that the susceptibility of the host allows the germs to gain a foothold.

3. THE NEWTONIAN MECHANICAL/CHEMICAL view of life vs the energy wave form view of life. The medical scientists insist that a human being consists mainly of flesh and bone which is altered by chemical processes. The natural fraternity maintain that energy waves manifest as physical humans.

4. THE REDUCTIONIST vs the holistic approach to physics. (Descartes vs Einstein). The medical scientists seek to investigate smaller and smaller components of matter whilst the natural researchers strive to look at the bigger and bigger picture.

5. MANAGEMENT of disease vs restoration of health. Medical scientists focus on fighting the disease while natural healers direct efforts at the causes, hoping to restore health.

6. THE EXCLUSION OF NON-MEASURABLES, from human health, by medical science. Medical models do not include items that cannot be measured such as love, beauty and justice. The natural models include these items inspite of the fact that they cannot be measured.

7. REJECTION of God from science vs inclusion of God in science. Medical science maintains a health model outside of Scripture. Natural healers include God in their health model.

IF THE MEDICAL industry professional has been saved, Scriptural arguments will make sense to him, but the professional side of his life is still possessed by Satan. This book should assist in the process of seeing the deception, in the mind of the saved medical industry professional.

CHAPTER 11
PROTECTING HEALTH

The two faces of protecting health are, MAINTAINING health and RESTORING health.

MAINTAINING HEALTH:
Health cannot be maintained outside of the dictates of God.

"AND SAID, if thou wilt diligently hearken to the voice of the Lord thy God, and wilt do that which is right in his sight, and wilt give ear to his commandments, and keep <u>all his statutes</u>, I will put <u>none</u> of these <u>diseases</u> upon thee, which I have brought upon the Egyptians, for I am the Lord that <u>healeth</u> thee." (Exodus 15:26)

THE SPIRIT of a human is the first priority to be considered for healing. The end of this chapter will include the simple advice on how to heal one's spirit. The decisions one takes around the healing of one's spirit, are for eternity. There is no point in having a sick spirit inside a healthy body! Therefore spiritual healing is a first priority.

Once one's spirit is healed, the soul (mind) can be renewed, as a second priority, by a process of dying to self, as explained by Paul.

"And be not conformed to this world: but <u>be ye transformed by the renewing of your mind</u>, that ye may prove what is that good, and acceptable, and perfect, will of God." (Romans 12:2. (KJV)).

There is also no point in having a perverted mind in a healthy body! Therefore healing of the mind is the second priority.

But, alas, the human body is mortal and subject to all the vagaries of malfunction and disease that have distressed humans for millennia. God created the mysterious and wonderful "life" which manifests as living bodies. God also created the boundaries within which these bodies may function. If the body transgresses these boundaries, it will malfunction, in spite of being spiritually saved; in spite of having a renewed mind. Where are the limits of these boundaries? No one knows them all, but some of the limits are evident from Scripture, as well as research, experience, anecdote and experimentation.

Healing of the body becomes the third priority. Physical health is not a prerequisite for salvation. Physical well-being is of importance whilst in this world. A sick body is however, a burden, and it would be prudent to treat one's body honorably whilst on earth.

At the very basis of the physical limits are, firstly NUTRITION, and secondly, POISON. Simple, as only the elegance of God can be. Fortunately humans are robust creatures and can easily withstand short periods (measured in weeks) of malnutrition and/or poisoning. Humans can even survive long periods of mild malnutrition and/or mild poisoning, but they then suffer disease and malfunction, exactly what is increasingly and disastrously happening worldwide. Waiting in the wings are hordes of salivating, ravenous, scheming "problem solvers", preying on the sick mass of humans, each healer offering slick solutions for body, mind and spirit. The medical industry must rank near the top of these repugnant "problem solvers".

DEMONIC AND PSYCHOSOMATIC symptoms are not considered at this point since spiritual and mind healing should already be taken care of before turning attention to the body.

BY ATTEMPTING healing in any other order than 1) Spiritual; 2) Mind: 3) Body; one risks a confusion of multiple symptoms which originate from all 3 causes. The 3 causes can present identical physical symptoms, for instance depression could be demonic, mind driven or organic, as can most other diseases.

NUTRITION

Nutrition is the most basic requirement for bodily health maintenance, as planned by God. Step one is to provide one's body with a regular supply of ALL the nutrients planned by God.

DR. WALLACH (ANIMAL and human pathologist), states in his audio tape entitled "Dead Doctor's don't Lie", that laboratory rats are fed at least 90 nutrients (because there is big money at stake in laboratory tests and the rats have to be ultra healthy); battery chickens are fed 23 nutrients (because they only have to live for 42 days); and human babies are fed approximately 21 nutrients in "scientific religion" formula milk (because there is big money at stake in sick babies and even more money when they grow into sick adults). He explains that with only 21 nutrients in their food, the infants will stay sick and alive.

BY EATING the processed food produced by the food industry, one has a ZERO possibility of obtaining all the required nutrients. Not only that, but the nutrients will be damaged, rearranged, irradiated, homogenized, treated, maltreated, chemicalized, heated, altered and generally perverted. The learned professors at the dietetics faculty whorehouses will solemnly declare that the food produced by their bosses (the food industry) is "adequate" to maintain human health. (The Scriptural connotation of whoring with the world is used here and not the sexual connotation).

The only way by which one has a remote chance of obtaining adequate nutrients, is to rely on organically produced food, failing which, to supplement with organic food extracts, failing which, to supplement with synthetic food supplements, in that order, or a combination of the three. Since it is a technical subject, one will have to glean information from knowledgeable people, or good literature which now abounds. Beware, the nutrient supplement industry is also infested with a large cadre of greedy crooks.

Some of the most respected nutritional authors are (and there are many, outside of the medical industry):

Dr. Jeffrey Bland
    Dr. Patrick Holford
    Dr. Michael Colgan
    Dr. Walter Veith
    Dr. Richard Kunin
    Dr. Francisco Contreras

They have various philosophical persuasions, but they have seen the nutrient light, and have conducted "real" research and have not stooped to whorish compromise with Big Business.

Poison #1

God created the human body with a "waste disposal system" characterized by phenomenal capabilities of protection against poison. One merely has to observe the typical hard drinking, heavy smoking individual, to marvel at the phenomenon whereby the person can survive such a daily onslaught for decades before succumbing to general breakdown. The biochemical processes (of which very few are well understood) act to remove the poisons from one's body, work by first detecting the offensive substance, and secondly, invoking one or more of the many detoxification processes. The poisonous substances created by God, including alcohol, have inerrant ways of warning the body about the inherent danger, including such signals as offensive taste, offensive odor, resonance of subatomic properties. The poisons which have been put in the food by God, such as plant or "phyto-" chemicals, possess self-limiting dangers, moderating factors and elegant detection markers; (or "checks and balances" in accounting language). Pharmacologists, of the "scientific religion" variety, have a sinister "mind block" when confronted with this beautiful evidence of how elegantly God's creation works when NOT interfered with.

WHEN PERVERTED MAN, especially the "scientific religion" variety, creates poisons, the built-in safeguards created by God are transcended, the boundaries crossed, the limits exceeded. The result is systematic, mass poisoning of the humans and all the other living systems, including the air, on and around the earth. The poisons have permeated the water, air, cosmetics, food, clothes, work places and homes.

SYNTHETIC HORMONES, heavy metals, radioactivity, hundreds of thousands of new chemicals, genetically engineered DNA and thousands of synthetic medicines are produced aggressively, loudly applauded by the "scientific religion" industries. These poisons have broken God's rules. The only way to avoid the dangers posed by these stealthy poisons is education. The mass produced doctors will not have a clue since they are a major part of the threat, and would shoot themselves in the foot if they had to start thinking about poisons. Fortunately, dedicated researchers have published their findings, for all to see. Beware – the New World Order is exploiting some of these dangers in order to implement global eco-fanatical awareness.

SOME OF THE worst poisons have been generated in the Godless, abusive and cruel animal products industry. Insane "scientific religion" scientists have rearranged the way God created animals, to "improve" production. By stuffing the suffering creatures with growth hormones, antibiotic concoctions, slime riddled poultry brains and contaminated offal from abattoirs, massive pools of

Frankenstein like microbe mutations are generated. To further pervert God's plans, the bones, blood, excrement, brains and heads are "recycled" back into animal feed, thereby turning herbivores into carnivores, and multiplying the pool of poisons geometrically. Mad cow's disease (JCD) has now permeated the global pool of animal feeds, spread by a strange protein-like particle called a "prion" which can grow readily in the brains of all mammals. Animals tend to concentrate poisons up to 1 million times more than plants do. To eat ANYTHING out of this cesspool of iniquity is perilous and can only lead to disease.

Poison #2

All intracellular and chemical transactions in the biochemical processes of life are conducted with minute electrical charges or polarities, small pluses and minuses which literally mean the difference between life and death. The reader has probably seen chemicals denoted with NA^+, CH^-, H^+, Cl^- or perhaps heard of the word "ion". These are but the tip of the "energetic wave form" iceberg created by the WORD of God. The stabilizing factor which holds the global mass in electrical orderliness, is the magnetic field of the earth. It resonates at the perfect resonant frequency, or rather, it was perfect until quite recently. Any interference in this field will WRECK the order, at the level of the atom, and at the resonance level of life.

Some of the most disruptive influences arise from radio transmitters, power lines, cellular phones, hair dryers, TV sets, electric blankets, computer VDT's, fluorescent lights, electric clocks, microwave ovens, cordless telephones and motor car alternators. Particularly powerful, the municipal power grids and metal redistribution boxes dotted around suburbia, have adversely influenced the health of billions of people. Mass housing for poor people is worst hit because of the proximity of overhead power lines.

There are many devices available which offer protection against electronic pollution: such as personal apparatus, home devices and also devices to reduce the electro-pollution at the source, for example on the cellular phone . The pollution can be measured by means of sensitive instrumentation.

Experts keep a low profile , mainly because of the snide comments directed at them by the "scientific religion" defenders. (Beware the esoteric vultures hawking clap trap gadgetry).

RESTORING HEALTH:

Instead of being custodians of our health, the medical industry persecutes innovative healers and healing products. It is patently obvious that no human errors are to blame, simply that Satan has highjacked the medical industry 'en masse'.

ONCE HEALTH IS LOST, to a greater or lesser extent, restoration of health revolves around reversing the slide, which progressed to the point where loss of health occurred. It would normally mean retracing the road which lead to the current status, albeit on a "fast rewind". A broad guideline is that it can take approximately one month of healing for every year which was spent in deterioration.

GOD HAS CREATED humans with the capacity to heal dramatically, as can be observed when cuts and bruises knit spontaneously, or where broken bones miraculously mend. There are simple pre-conditions to healing, namely that the causes of, or obstructions to, the healing process be:

IDENTIFIED, and Removed or reduced, and optionally Employing a therapy to accelerate the removal and/or healing process.

THE PROBABLE CAUSES have been explained in this chapter. Once one's health is compromised, one's body may become microbe and parasite infested. These conditions may require some special clearing processes, best left to experienced health practitioners.

Unless the correct nutrients are provided and the resident poisons are removed, the healing process will be compromised.

Many formerly ill people have embarked on a "do-it-yourself" program, and with great success. Others prefer to employ external help in the form of professional healers, therapists or specialists such as test centers or pathologists. Very ill people often benefit from "farming" out their disease to an array of people, simultaneously or sequentially.

The more knowledge the health practitioner has, and the more modalities he or she is familiar with, the better the healing process will be. Specialists are dangerous since they tend to develop tunnel vision and myopic attitudes. Only high technology requires a specialist, such as an eye surgeon. Beware: specialists sell their speciality! An ENT (ear nose and throat) specialist is almost sure to advise sinus surgery for a blocked nose caused by colon candida (mould overgrowth in the colon). Beware: The world of natural health practitioners is riddled with charlatans, freaks, new age gurus and rip-off artists.

The author has found that a team consisting of a nutritional/energy specialist plus an ex medical-doctor-converted-to natural healing, can attend to most healing issues.

Listed below are some modest as well as very powerful non-medical therapies. (Abridged from Dr. Wilner's book).

The therapies share certain characteristics namely: they deal with the cause; promote normal processes; if toxic substances are used in the therapy it is of the God made variety.

BEWARE: some of these therapies are marginally dangerous and require the help of skilled health practitioners.

The choice therapies have been indicated as follows:

** = PRIME THERAPIES.
 * = good choice.

SAFE AND EFFECTIVE THERAPIES THAT MAKE SENSE:

Amygdalin**. (variations: Vitamin B17, Laetrile and Proanthocyanidin). Used as antioxidants.

CHELATION**. (EDTA IV is the most popular). To remove plaque from arteries.

THE BREATH OF LIFE (Air in many forms):
 Ozone**
 Oxygen**
 Cryogenic Cell Therapy
 DMSO*
 Hydrogenperoxide**
 Magnesiumperoxide**
 Nascent oxygen**

"LET YOUR FOOD BE YOUR MEDICINE" (Medicine from the plant world)

LINSEED, The Incredible Oil **

THE BUDWIG THERAPY*

NATURE'S FOOD MEDICINES:
- Garlic
- Green Tea*
- MSM
- Enzyme Therapy**
- Digestive Enzymes*
- Onconase*
- Enzyme Preparations

VITAMINS AND MINERALS:
- All of them

WHEN THE PEOPLE FIGHT BACK - VICTORY! (Canadian health battle)

714 - X* (Nitroamoniocamphor)

UNIVERSAL ENERGY:
- Electromagnetic Therapies
- Electromagnetic Field Therapy
- Neuroprobe
- T.E.N.S
- Phototherapy
- Tachyon Energy - Pulsors.
- Hyperthermia
- Ions

SUGGESTED NUTRITIONAL SUPPLEMENTS:
- Algae
- Spirulina
- Chlorella
- Bugula
- Amino Acids*

Bee Pollen
Benzaldehyde*
Cabbage (Indoles)*
Canthaxanthin*
Chlorophyll
DHEA*
Essential Fatty Acids
Evening Primrose Oil
Fibre*
Herbs
Aloe *
Astragalus
Mistletoe
Herbal Formulas
Glandular and Nerve Tonic
Ayurvedic Herbal Medicines
Chaparral
Chinese Herbal Medicine**
Ginseng
The Essiac Formula**
Ubiquinone (Co-Enzyme Q-10)

LET YOUR MEDICINE BE YOUR FOOD (Use these for everyday cooking):
Mushrooms**
Kombucha*
Maitake
Reishi
Shiitake
P'au D'Arco Tea*
Seaweed
Spices

OTHER SIGNIFICANT THERAPIES:
Anti-Neoplastons (Dr. Burzinski)
Cancell*

Carnivora
Colon Cleansing*
Alimentary (digestive tract) Toxemias
Gerson Therapy
Glandulars*
Hoxsey Therapy
Hydrazine Sulphate
IAT (Immuno-augmentative Therapy)
Koch Therapy
Livingston Therapy

IMMUNE STIMULANTS:
Aristolochia Acid
Bestatin
Coley's toxins
Gossypol
Inosine
Krestin
Lentinan
Levamisol
Methylene Blue
Monoclonal Antibodies
MTH-68
Muroctasin
Shark Cartilage
SOD
Splenopentin
Vaccines - BCG, Staphage Lysate, Maruyama
Urea

OTHER PRODUCTS TO CONSIDER - MAYBE!
Not natural, Not safe. Medical industry drugs! Useful, but ultra-toxic.

ANTICOAGULANTS - WARFARIN

Heparin
Nafazatron
Aspirin
Flutamide
Megace
Tamoxifen
Thioproline

"Behold, I stand at the door, and knock: if any man hear my voice, and open the door, I will come in to him, and will sup with him, and he with me. (Revelations 3:20." (KJV)).

References:
1. Exodus 15:26. (KJV).
2. Romans 12:2. (KJV).
3. Revelations 3:20.(KJV).
4. Veith, Dr. Walter. *Diet and Health, new scientific perspectives.* (1991).
5. Cannon, Geoffrey. *Superbug, nature's revenge.* (1995).
6. Webb, Tony and Lang, Tim. *Food Irradiation.* (1990).
7. Blythman, Joanna. *The Food We Eat.* (1996).
8. Davis, Dr. Karen. *Prisoned Chickens, Poisoned Eggs.* (1996).
9. Oski, Frank A. *Don't drink your Milk!* (1996).
10. Rifkin, Jeremy. *Beyond Beef.* (1992).
11. Gellatley, Juliet. *The Silent Ark.* (1996).
12. Colborn, Dr. Theo. *Our Stolen Future.* (1996).
13. Perucca, Fabien and Pouradier, Gerard. *The Rubbish on our Plates.* (1996).
14. Cox, Peter and Brusseau. *Secret Ingredients.* (1997).
15. Becker, Dr. Robert O. *Cross Currents.* (1990).
16. Davidson, Dr. John. *The Web of Life.* (1988).
17. Coats, Callum. *Living Energies.* (1996).
18. Willner, Dr. Robert E. *The cancer Solution.* (1994).

GLOSSARY OF TERMS AND CONCEPTS

Agonist Refers to nutrient interactions which promote one another.

Allopathic The approach of treating disease by suppressing symptoms eg. anti-spasmodic, anti-biotic etc.

Amino acid Building blocks of protein that consist of amino basic group (nitrogen & hydrogen) and acid of carboxyl group (carbon, oxygen and hydrogen)

Anecdotal Relating an event as seen or experienced.

Antagonist Refers to nutrient interactions that inhibit one another. Copper and zinc are antagonists (zinc inhibits copper absorption), while calcium and vitamin D are antagonists (vitamin D helps to promote calcium absorption).

Asclepius/aesclepia Symbol of the serpent wound around the staff of life.

Blood-brain barrier This is a cellular barrier which prevents certain chemicals from passing from the blood to the brain. Many amino acids and substances are blocked from entering into the brain readily without transport system.

Catecholamine An adlrenaline-like substance in the brain - norepinephrine, epinephrine and dopamine, which is made from tyrosine.

Chiropractic Healing art centered around the manipulation of the spinal column.

Codex Alimentarius Standards set in order to regulate global food trade.

Cofactor The part of an enzyme that is usually a mineral or trace metal important for the activity of the enzyme.

Covalent bond A type of bond between molecules which is not polarized or electric

D, L and DL Amino acids occur in D and L forms. The D form rotates light to the right, while the L form rotates to the left. When the amino acid occurs in DL, it's a mixture of D and L.

Demonisation The influence of demons upon a portion of a human activity.

Demon oppression The stronghold of demons upon a portion of a human activity.

Demon possession The ownership of demons upon a portion of a human activity.

Dogma Inflexible opinion.

Double-blind placebo controlled crossover study The statistical testing processes whereby the placebo effect (mind-over-body-influence) is eliminated.

Double-blind study A study in which neither doctors or patients are clear as to who is getting the medicine and who's getting the placebo or non-medicine. This method is used statistically to identify successful treatments.

Elemental medicine Those healing arts which are directed at the basics of the life form, (before energy becomes matter) as opposed to the treatment of the physical dimension only.

Enzymes Very large protein that activate certain reactions in the body to form specific substances.

Ethnomedicine Medicine which has been developed by an ethnic group over time.

Eugenics The deliberate manipulation of human breeding in order to influence the composition of a race. It includes abortion, birth control and selective pairing.

Fatty acid An acid derived from the series of open chain hydrocarbons, usually obtained from the saponification of fats.

Genocide The eradication by death of large groups of humans.

Gnosticism Knowledge which is not shared, but used to obtain power.

Inotrope A drug or nutrient that promotes the pumping action of the heart, i.e., calcium, taurine or digoxin.

In vitro A Latin term for studies done in tent tubes.

GLOSSARY OF TERMS AND CONCEPTS

Krebs cycle Famous metabolic cycle discovered by Hans Krebs of England, a Nobel prizewinner. This refers to the metabolic pathway in which carhohydrates are broken down into energy.

Loading An experimental process in which one element or nutrient is given in extremely large doses to overload the system and then to study its effect.

Metabolite A product or part of a metabolic pathway.

Metabolic pathway The way in which energy is taken from protein, fat or carbohydrate. There are thousands of metabolic pathways in the body. The main ones are carbohydrate (Krebs) and fatty acid. Protein mainly uses the carbohydrate pathway.

Molecule A minute mass of matter; smallest quantity into which a substance can be divided and retain its characteristic properties.

Neurotransmitter These are often made up of amino acids or peptides and refer to chemical languages by which cells (neurons) of the brain communicate with each other. As we speak different languages, so do cells speak to each other in different languages.

New Age Belief system whereby the destiny of mankind is directed by mass human endeavour.

NPU (net protein utilization) The way in which protein is utilized. Some foods contain protein that cannot be metabolized adequately.

Necromancy Deliberate tampering with a corpse.

Occultic Secular activities which centre around fields of knowledge outside of Scripture and standard human practice.

Osteopathy Healing art centered around the manipulation of the skull.

Oxidation The burning of fuel to supply energy in the body.

Peptide A link between two amino acids. Peptide refers to two or more amino acids.

Pharmaceutical/medical/industrial/complex The overlap and joint efforts of diverse industries acting in concert.

Phospholipid substance consisting primarily of fatty acids and phosphorus, such as lecithin, occurring in all membranes.

Precursor Refers to a previous product, for example, the precursor of a cake is its ingredients.

Protein A collection of amino acids. Protein is one of the building blocks of the body. Others are fat, carbohydrates, and minerals.

Psychotropic drugs Drugs that affect the mind and the psychology of an individual.

Reductionism Philosophy whereby a subject, or matter, is studied by reducing it to its smallest possible components

Reincarnational Healing purportedly directed at previous life or lives of the patient.

Reprobate mind A biblical concept denoting a mind so corrupt that it drives the person to perform loathsome activities.

Ritual Elaborate procedure performed before engaging in a repetitive event. .

Serial deception Repetitive deception of the same group, by the same group, on the same subject.

Serotonin A major neurotransmitter in the brain made from tryptophan

Shamanism Mystic powers of healing and insight endowed to the shaman (witchdoctor) of a tribe of (normally primitive) peopl

Tachyon Popular health use of materials which vibrate beyond the classical physics boundaries, even faster than the speed of light.

Telencephalic A portion of the lower brain that develops into olfactory lobes, cerebral cortex, and corpora striata.

Urea cycle A particular metabolic pathway metabolizing the urea. It is cyclical in nature and always ends up discarding the urea.

Vasopressin A type of hormone (also known as anti-diuretic hormone) that may be useful to memory.

INDEX

Academic
- ADA
- Aids
- Allopathic
- Alternative
- AMA
- Ambulance
- American Dietetic Association
- American Medical Association
- Anecdatal
- Antibiotics
- Associations
- Asthma
- Babies
- BASF
- Bayer
- Belief system
- Bible
- Biochemical
- Blame
- Blood pressure

Brain
Bristol=Myers
Business
Caduceus
Cancer
Carnegie
Cartel
Cell
Cellular-medicine
Charm
Chemicals
Chlorine
Cholesterol
Christian
Christian
Church
Clinical
Codex Alimentarius
Control
Coronary heart disease
Council
Creation
Crimes
Cross
Crossover study
Curse
Death
Deceiver
Depression
Dietetics
Disease
Disease
Divination
Divination
Divine
DNA
Double-blind

Dragon
Drug.
Drugs
DuBois-Raymond
Dynamics
Efficacy
Electrical force
Electricity
Electromagnetism
Emotions
Energetic
Energy
Enzymes
Epilepsy
Erasistratus
Ethnomedicine
Ethno-piracy
Eugenics
Evil
Evolution
Farben
Fellowships
Female
Fertility
Food
Forces
Forces
Foundation
Francis Bacon
Frankenstein, dr
Fraud
Galen
Genetic
Genocide
Germs
Glaxo/Wellcome
God

Government
Gunther Rexrodt
Hahnemann
Healer
Healing
Health
Health care
Health insurance
Heart disease
Helmut Kohl
Herb
Hippocrates
Hippocratic oath
Hoechst
Holistic
Holistic
Holy spirit
Homeopathic
Honesty
Hormones
Hormones
Horoscope
Horst Seehofer
Horus
Hospitals
Humanity
Hypertension
Hypothesis
Idiopathic
Idolatry
Illegal
Illegal
Immortality
Immunity
Industry
Infection
Infection

INDEX

Infectious diseases
Infertility
Insanity
Institutions
Integrative
Johannes Kepler
Julius Bernstein
Justice
Keykeion
Legislation
Life
Life force
Logo
Louis XVI
Luigi Galvani
Magic
Magnet Therapy
Magnetism
Magnetism
Manfred Kanther
Masonic
Mechanists
Medical
Medical aid
Medical Industry
Medicine
Mental
Merck
Mesmer
Mortality
Mothers
Muslim
Mutation
Mystic
Mysticism
Myth
Natural

Naturopathic
Necromancy
Neurosis
New Age
Newton
Nicolas Copernicus
Nikola Testa
Norvatis
Nutrients
Nutrition
Oath
Occultic
Occultism
Old Testament
Optimal
Orthodox
Otto Lowei
Paracelsus
Paradigm
Paramedical
Pathogen
Pathology
Patients
Paul Ehrlich
Pendulums
Pfiser
Pharmaceutical
Pharmacology
Pharm-med-ind complex
Philosophy
Physicians
Physicists
Placebo
Poison
Priest
Probiotics
Profession

Prognostication
Propaganda
Prostitutes
Psychobabble
Psychoheresy
Psycho-industry
Psychology
Psychoseduction
Psychostimulants
Radiation
Radio-activity
Rath, dr Matthias
Religion
Religion
Rene` Descartes
Research
Resonance
Rhone-Poulenc-Rhorer
Ritalin
Roche
Rockefeller
Rothschilds
Rx
Sacred
Safety
Salvation
Satan
Schools
Science
Scripture
Selection
Self-esteem
Semmelweiss, dr
Serpent
Serpent
Sin
Soothsaying

Sorcery
Specialists
Stool
Strategy
Superbugs
Supplements
Surgery
Synthetic
Tachyon
Technology
Temole
Tests
Theology
Therapists
Thomas Edison
Toxic
Traditional
Treatment
Tribunal
Triumvirate
Truth
Unbeliever
Universities
Vaccination
Victim
VIRUS
Vitalist
Vitamins
Water
Wellbeing
Western medicine
White
WHO
FAO
Pharma-cartel
William Gilbert
Wisdom

Witchcraft
Witchcraft
Witches
Wizardry
Woman
Wonder

REFERENCE

References to Scripture are taken from the Authorized King James Version of the Holy Bible unless otherwise stated.

Dakes Annotated Reference Bible. (KJV) (1993):

D.B.S. Inc. Lawrenceville, Georgia, U.S.A. p 566 column 4 note g; p 80 column 4 note f; p 75 column 1 note b.

Hoffman, Dr. Jay M. (1979): Hunza, 15 Secrets of the world's healthiest and oldest living People.

Professional Press Publishing, Valley Center, U S A.

McMillen Dr. S. I.(1994): None of these Diseases.

Baker Book House Company, Grand Rapids, Michigan, U S A

Brand, Dr. Paul and Philip Yancey.(1987):
Fearfully and wonderfully made.
Zondervan Books, Grand Rapids, Michigan, U S A

Pauling, Linus.(1987): How to live longer and feel better.

Avon Books, New York. U S A

Grossinger, Dr. Richard. (1995): Planet Medicine Modalities.

North Atlantic Books, Berkeley, U S A

Becker, Dr. Robert O. (1985):The Body Electric.

Quill, New York, U S A p 331

Schauberger, Victor. (Translated by Callum Coates) (1998):

The Water Wizard. Gateway Books, Bath , U K p 46-52

Altman, Nathanial. (1995): Oxygen healing Therapies.

Healing Arts Press, Rochester, U S A p 28-30 Viebahn, Dr. Renate. (1994): The use of Ozone in Medicine. Haug, Heidelberg, Germany p 16-17

REFERENCE

Becker, Dr. Robert O. (1990): Cross Currents. G.P. Putnam's Sons, New York, U S A p 13-26

Capra, Dr. Fritjof. (1983): The turning Point.
 Harper Collins Publishers, London, U K p 28

Udo Becker. (1994): Encyclopedia of Symbols.

Element Books, Dorset, U K p 164

Hunt, Dave. (1996): In defense of Faith.
 Harvest House Publishers, Eugene, U S A
 p 213-215

Otto, Dr. L Bettman. (1956): A pictorial History of Medicine. Charles C. Thomas Publishing, U S A p 91

Calder, Ritchie. (1958): Medicine and Man.
 C. Tinling & Co. London, U K p 57

Strong, Dr. James. (1995): Exhaustive Concordance of the Bible. Thomas Nelson Publishers, London, U K p 95 (Greek)

Randles, Pastor Bill. (1996): Making War in the Heavenlies. St Matthew Publications, Cambridge, U K p 90-98

Comfort, Ray. (1989): Hell's best kept Secret.
 Living Waters Publications, Bellflower, U S A p 19-26

Murphy, Dr. Ed. (1996): The Handbook for spiritual Warfare. Thomas Nelson Publishers, Nashville, U S A p 27

Hislop, Rev. Alexander. (1916): The Two Babylons.
   LoiZeaux Brothers, Neptune, U S A

Kushi, Michio. (1978): Natural healing through Macrobiotics. Japan Publications, New York, U S A p 8

Hunt, Dave. (1994): A Woman rides the Beast.
   Harper Collins Publishers, London, U K

Griffen, G. Edward. (1978): World without Cancer.

American Media, Westlake Village, U S A

Morris Fishbein, M.D.A. (1947) History of the A M A. (American Medical Association.)

W.B. Saunders. Co. Philadelphia & London, p 987, 989

Goulden, Joseph. (1971): The Money Givers.

Random House, New York

Morris, A. Bealle. (1958): The new Drug Story.
Columbia Publishing Co. Washington, D.C.
p 19, 20

Moss, Dr. Ralph W. (1996): The Cancer Industry.
Equinox Press, New York, U S A p 392

McAlvany, Donald S. (1997): The McAlvany Intelligence Advisor. Phoenix, U S A November issue, p 17

Hunt, Dave. (1998): Occult Invasion.

Harvest House Publishers, Eugene, U S A

Icke, Dave. (1997): And the Truth shall set you free. Bridge of Love publications, London

Hunt, Dave. (1985): The seduction of Christianity.

Harvest House Publishers, Eugene, U S A
   McAlvany, Donald S. (1997): The McAlvany Intelligence Advisor. Phoenix , U S A, November issue, p 17

Oden, Rev. Clifford. (1976): Thank God I have Cancer. Arlington House, New York U S A p 90-92

Veith, Dr. Walter. (1993): Diet and Health, new scientific Perspectives. Southern Publishing Association, Cape Town, South Africa

REFERENCE

Collins (1984): Collins compact Dictionary of the English Language. Wm. Collins & Sons, London

Dufty, William. (1975): Sugar Blues.

Warner Books, New York, U S A p 93
    Marrs, Texe.(1989): Mega Forces.

Living Truth Publishers, Austin, U S A

Capra, Dr. Fritjof. (1983)The turning Point.

Harper Collins Publishers, London, U K p 37-52

Milton, Richard. (1993): The facts of Life. Shattering the Myths of Darwinism.

Corgi Books, London, U K

Taylor, Ian T. (1991):In the Minds of Men : Darwin and the New World Order. T F E Publishing, Toronto, Canada

Colborn, Theo. (1997): Our stolen Future. Abacus, London, U K

Chetley, Andrew. (1995): Problem Drugs.

Zeal Books, London, U K p 3

Goodman, Rall, Nies and Taylor. (1992): The pharmacological Basis of Therapeutics. McGraw Hill, New York, U S A

Graedon, Joe and Teresa. (1995): Deadly Drug Interactions. St Martin's Press, New York, U S A

Melville, Arabella. (1982): Cured to Death.

Nel Books, London, U K

Cain, Miriam. (1995): Fight for Life. African Christian Action, Glosderry, South Africa

CAFMR newsletter. (Spring 1996). Campaign against fraudulent medical Research, Lawson, Australia (www.pnc.com.au/~cafmr.)

McTaggart, Lynne. (1996): What Doctors don't tell you. Harper Collins Publishers, London, U K.

Deparrie, Paul & Pride, Mary. (1988): Unholy Sacrifices of the new Age. Crossway Books, Westchester, U S A p 122-125

Mendelsohn, Dr. Robert S.(1984): How to raise a healthy Child in spite of your Doctor. Ballantine Books, New York, U S A

Contreras, Dr. Francisco. (1997): Health in the 21st Century. Interpacific Press, Chula Vista, U S A

Mendelsohn, Dr. Robert S.(1982): Mal(e) Practice - how Doctors manipulate Women. Contemporary Books, Chicago, U S A p 150-156

Colgan, Dr. Michael.(1993): Optimum Sports Nutrition. Advanced Research Press, Ronkonkoma, U S A p 249-253

Wan Ho, Dr. Mae. (1998):Genetic Engineering.

Gateway Books, Bath, U K p 14

McKenna, Dr. John. (1996): Alternatives to Antibiotics. Struik Publishers, Cape Town, South Africa

Cannon, Geoffrey. (1995): Superbug.

Virgin Publishing, London, U K

Miller, Neil Z . (1996): Immunization – Theory vs Reality. New Atlantean Press, Santa Fe, New Mexico

Brand, Dr. Paul and Philip Yancey. (1987): Fearfully and wonderfully made. Zondervan Books, Grand Rapids, U S A

Breggin. Dr. Peter. (1993): Toxic Psychiatry, An all-out Attack against the

Deception. Harper Collins, London U K p 378

Chetley, Andrew.(1995): Problem Drugs. Zeal Books, London, U K p 204-209

Contreras, Dr. Francisco. (1997): Health in the 21st Century. Interpacific Press, Chula Vista, U S A

Yiamouyiannis, Dr. John. (1995): Aids. Health Action Press, Delaware, U S A

McTaggart, Lynne. (1996): What Doctors don't tell you. Harper Collins Publishers, London, U K

Carter, Dr. James P. (1992): Racketeering in Medicine. Hampton Roads Publishing, Norfolk, U S A

Goodman, Rall, Nies and Taylor. (1992): The pharmacological Basis of Therapeutics. McGraw Hill, New York, U S A p 405-414

Thompson, Stuart (1998): Pharmapact. (People's Health Alliance Rejecting Medical Authoritarianism And Conspiratorial Tyranny). South Africa

Laurence, Leslie and Weinhouse, Beth. (1994): Outrageous Practices. Ballantine Books, New York, U S A

1. Moss, Dr. Ralph W. (1996): The Cancer Industry. Equinox Press, New York, U S A p VIII.
2. Willner, Dr. Robert E. (1994): The Cancer Solution. Peltec Publishing, Boca Raton, U S A p III

3. Dermer, Dr. Gerald B. (1994): The immortal Cell. Avery, New York, U S A

Goldberg, Burton. (1997): Cancer. Future Medicine Publishing, Tiburon, U S A

Epperson, Ralph A. (1985): The unseen Hand. Publius Press, Tucson, U S A p 37, quoting Nesta Webster

Willner, Dr. Robert E.(1994): Deadly Deception.(Dust Cover). Peltec Publishing, Boca Raton, U S A

Duesburg, Dr. Peter H. (1996): AIDS: Virus or Drug induced? Contemporary Issues in Genetics and Evolution. Kluver Academic Publishers, London, U K

Shenton, Joan. (1998): Positively false: Exposing the Myth around HIV and Aids. S E Martins Press, New York, U S A

Rath, Dr. Matthias. (1993): Eradicating Heart Disease. Health Now, San Francisco, U S A p 10-11

Moore, Dr. Richard D. (1993): The high Blood Pressure Solution. Healing Arts Press, Rochester, U S A

McCully, Dr. Kilmer S. (1997): The Homocysteine Revolution. Keats Publishing, New Canaan, U S A

Hunt, Dave. (1996): In Defense of the Faith. Harvest House Publishers, Eugene, U S A p 204-205

Trull, Louise B. (1993): The CanCell Controversy. Hampton Roads Publishing, Norfolk, U S A

Schiff, Michel. (1994): The Memory of Water. Thorson's, London, U K

Alexanderson, Olof. (1997): Living Water. Victor Schauberger and the Secrets of natural Energy. Gateway Books, Bath, U K p 17

Bird, Christopher. (1990): The Persecution and Trial of Gaston Naessens. H. J. Kramer, Tiburon, U S A

Doyal, Lesley & Pennell, Imogen. (1979): The Political Economy of Health. Cromwell Press, Melksham, U K p 37

Benson, Ivor. (1986): The Zionist Factor. Veritas Publishing, Australia p 137

Simpson, William Gayley. (1978): Which Way western Man? National Alliance, Washington, U S A p 699-713

McAlvany, Donald S. (1997): The McAlvany Intelligence Advisor. November issue, Phoenix, U S A

IAHF.(1998): International Advocates for Health Freedom. U S A (http://www.iahf.com.)

A D A (American Dietetics Association) (1996): ADA Position Statement. Journal of American Dietetics Association, vol 96, no 1

The Life extension Foundation U S A (http://www.lef.org)

Carter, Dr. James P. (1992): Racketeering in Medicine. Hampton Roads Publishing, Norfolk, U S A p 190

Bobgan, Dr. Martin and Deidre.(1987): Psychoheresy. Psychoheresy Awareness Ministries, Santa Barbara, U S A

Szasz, Thomas. (1978): The Myth of Psychotherapy. Anchor/Doubleday, Garden City, p 25

Lasch, Christopher. (1979): The Culture of Narcissism. W W Norton & Company, Inc., New York, U S A

Torrey, Dr. E. Fuller. (1972): The Mind Game. Penquin, New York, p 8

Pfeiffer, Dr. Carl. (1987): Nutrition and Mental Illness. Healing Arts Press, Rochester, U S A

Breggin, Dr. Peter R. (1993): Toxic Psychiatry. Harper Collins, London, U K

Psychoheresy Awareness Ministeries. PAMSM (http://www.psychoheresy.aware.org)

Ripplinger, Gail A. (1993): New Age Bible Versions. A V Publications, Ararat, U S A p 101

Ash, David A. (1995): The New Science of the Spirit. The College of Psychic Studies, London, U K p 35

Coats, Callum. (1996): Living Energies. Gateway Books, Bath, U K p 36

Begich, Dr. Nick. (1995): Angels don't play this Haarp. Earthpulse Press, Anchorage, Alaska

Hislop, Alexander.(1959): The two Babylons. Loizeaux Brothers, Neptune U S A p 197-205

Hunt, Dave. (1988): Whatever happened to Heaven? Harvest House Publishers, Eugene, U S A p 113

Ankerberg, Dr. John and Weldon, Dr. John.(1996): Encyclopedia of New Age Beliefs. Harvest House Publishers, Eugene, U S A

Lewis, C. S. (19): The screwtape Letters. New York, Macmillan Publishing, 1980

Melville, Arabella. (1982): Cured to Death. Nel Books, London, U K p 205

Veith, Dr. Walter. (1991): Diet and Health, new scientific Perspectives. Southern Publishing Association, Cape Town, South Africa

Cannon, Geoffrey. (1995): Superbug, Nature's revenge. Virgin Publishing, London, U K

Webb, Tony and Lang, Tim. (1990): Food Irradiation. Thorsons, London, U K

Blythman, Joanna. (1996): The Food we eat.
 Michael Joseph, London, U K

Davis, Dr. Karen. (1996): Prisoned Chickens, Poisoned Eggs. Book Publishing, Summer Town, U S A

Oski, Frank A. (1996): Don't drink your Milk!
 Teach Services, New York, U S A

Rifkin, Jeremy. (1992): Beyond Beef. Plume, New York, U S A

Gellatley, Juliet. (1996): The silent Ark. Thorsons, London, U K

Colborn, Dr. Theo. (1996): Our stolen Future. Abacus, London, U K

Perucca, Fabien and Pouradier, Gerard.(1996): The Rubbish on our Plates. Prism Books, London, U K

Cox, Peter and Brusseau. (1997): Secret Ingredients. Bantam, London, UK

Becker, Dr. Robert O. (1990): Cross Currents.
 G.P. Putnam's Sons, New York, U S A

Davidson, Dr. John. (1988): The Web of Life.
C.W. Daniel, Essex, U K
Coats, Callum.(1996): Living Energies. Gateway Books, Bath, U K

Willner, Dr. Robert E. (1994): The Cancer Solution. Peltec Publishing, Boca Raton, U S A

Copyright © 2017 by Dr. Charl Du Randt

All rights reserved.

No part of this book may be reproduced in any form or by any electronic or mechanical means, including information storage and retrieval systems, without written permission from the author, except for the use of brief quotations in a book review.